# CLEAN PALEO
# FAMILY COOKBOOK

## Essentials to Get Started

### MELISSA TAYLOR

# TABLE OF CONTENTS

---- BREAKFAST ----

---- LUNCH ----

# Breakfast

# GINGER ZUCCHINI BREAD

Slice this bread and put it on a platter for a party, or serve it on Christmas morning. Either way, it's sure to be a big hit with all; no one will suspect it's actually healthy

MAKES 8 SERVING/ TOTAL TIME 1 HOUR

## INGREDIENTS

1 cup Almond flour

1/2 tsp Sea salt

2 tbsp Cinnamon

1 tbsp Ground ginger

2 tbsp Honey

1 tsp Ground cloves

1/2 tsp Baking soda

1/2 tsp Allspice

1/4 tsp Nutmeg

1 tsp Vanilla

1 Zucchini (small, grated)

3 Eggs

## METHOD

### STEP 1
Preheat oven to 350 degrees F.
Combine the almond flour, salt, baking soda, and spices in a bowl. In a separate bowl, mix the remaining ingredients. Whisk well and add to the dry.

### STEP 2
Brush a loaf pan with coconut oil or cooking spray. Pour the batter into the pan and bake for 40 to 50 minutes, until a toothpick inserted in the center comes out clean. Allow to cool before slicing.

**NUTRITION VALUE**

335 Kcal, 14g fat,
8g fiber, 32g protein, 15g carbs.

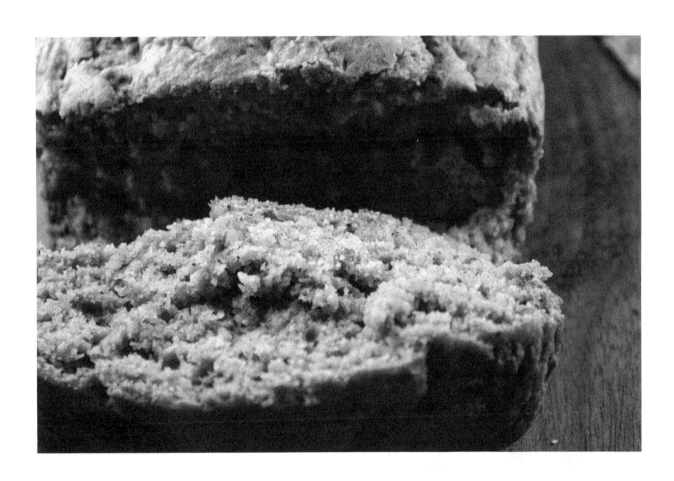

# PALEO CHILI LIME BROILED AVOCADO

Full of heart-healthy fat, broiled avocado is ultra-creamy and delicious.

MAKES 2 SERVING/ TOTAL TIME 10 MINUTE

## INGREDIENTS

1 Avocado (pitted)

1 tsp Honey

1 Lime (juiced)

1/2 tsp Chili powder

Sea salt (to taste)

## METHOD

**STEP 1**

Preheat broiler to high heat. Drizzle the avocado halves with the honey and lime juice.

Lay on a baking sheet and broil for 5-6 minutes, until avocado flesh begins to blister. Remove from oven and sprinkle with chili powder and salt. Serve warm.

## NUTRITION VALUE

625 Kcal, 20 fat,
11g fiber, 54.2g protein, 14 carbs.

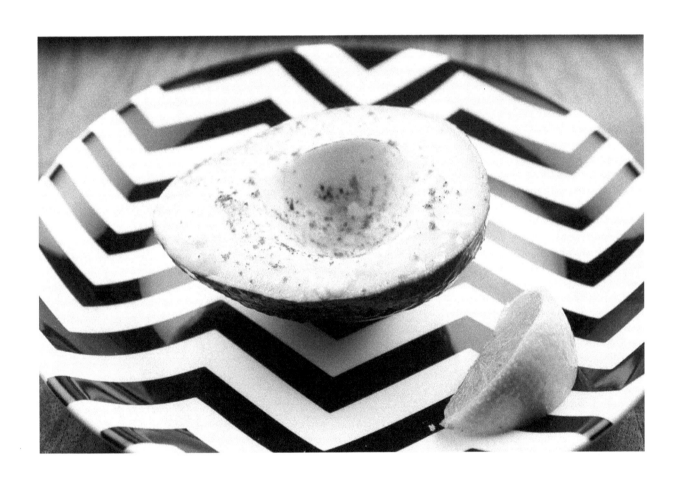

# CURRIED VEGETABLE SKILLET WITH FRIED EGGS

Curried vegetable skillet mixed with fried eggs sound so healthy and yummy.

MAKES 2 SERVING/ TOTAL TIME 15 MINUTE

## INGREDIENTS

4 tbsp olive oil

1 tbsp Curry powder

2 cups Baby spinach

2 Leeks (sliced)

1 Carrot (grated)

2 Garlic cloves (minced)

4 Eggs

Sea salt and fresh ground pepper (to taste)

## METHOD

### STEP 1

Heat half the oil in a large skillet. Add the vegetables and cook until soft. Stir in the curry powder, cook for an additional minute, and then turn off heat.

### STEP 2

Heat a nonstick skillet over medium high heat. Add the remaining oil and fry the eggs to your liking.
Serve the eggs on top of the vegetables.

| NUTRITION VALUE | 335 Kcal, 14g fat, 8g fiber, 32g protein, 15g carbs. |
|---|---|

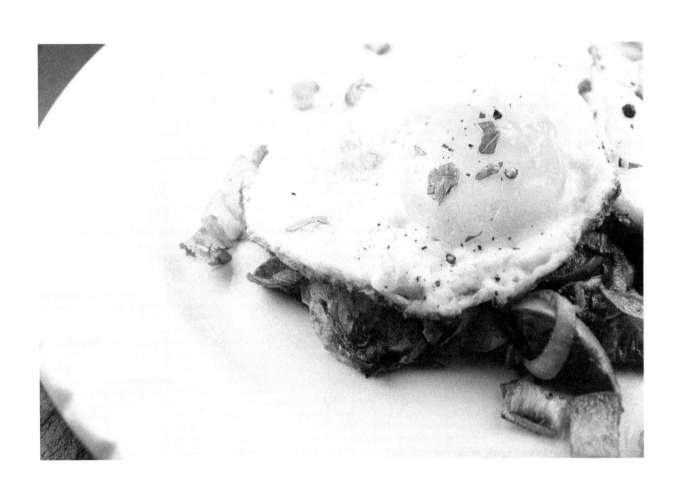

# EGG BAKED IN ACORN SQUASH

This recipe is an interesting twist on a classic Toad in the Hole.

MAKES 2 SERVING/ TOTAL TIME  1 HOUR

## INGREDIENTS

1 Acorn squash (cut in half and deseeded)

2 Eggs

1 tbsp Fresh chives (chopped)

Salt (to taste)

Black pepper (to taste)

## METHOD

### STEP 1

Preheat oven to 375 degrees F.

Place the squash face down on a baking sheet. Bake the squash in the oven for 25-35 minutes, until the squash becomes tender. Remove from the oven and allow to cool slightly, about 5 minutes.

### STEP 2

Place the squash halves face up on the baking sheet. Crack on egg into the hole in each half. Season with salt and pepper and bake in the oven for 15 to 20 minutes, until the egg sets.

Remove from the oven. Garnish with fresh chives and serve.

| NUTRITION  VALUE | 469 Kcal, 19g fat, 8g fiber, 45g protein, 14.9g carbs. |
|---|---|

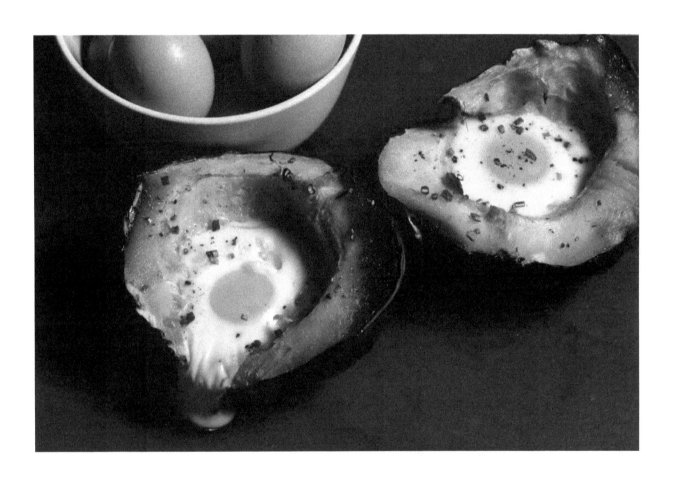

# AVOCADO EGG SALAD

Egg salad is one of the traditional salads that's rich in protein and full of flavor.

MAKES 1 SERVING/ TOTAL TIME 5 MINUTE

## INGREDIENTS

1 Egg (Hard-boiled)

1/2 Avocado (diced

2 slices bacon (crumbled)

Juice from ½ a lemon

Sea salt (to taste)

Black pepper (to taste)

## METHOD

**STEP 1**

Slightly mash the avocado. Drizzle with lemon juice.

Dice the hard-boiled egg and add it to the avocado.

Add the bacon, mix gently to combine. Season with sea salt and black pepper.

Serve immediately.

**NUTRITION VALUE**

224 Cal , 18g fat, 4g saturated fat, 5g fiber, 21g protein, 7g carbs.

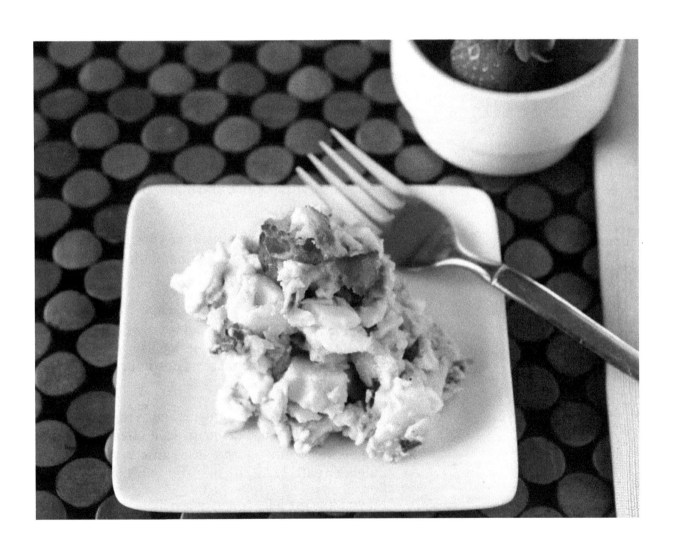

# PERFECT PALEO YOGURT

This simple recipe will have you stocking up on **yogurt** and storing it in the fridge to eat on the go during your morning commute!

MAKES 2 SERVING/ TOTAL TIME 10 MINUTE

## INGREDIENTS

1 can Coconut milk (about 2 c)

1 pack Gelatin (about 2 tbsp)

Juice from 1 lime (about 2 tbsp)

1/2 tsp Vanilla extract

1 tbsp Honey

Raisins (optional)

Cinnamon (optional)

Honey (optional)

## METHOD

Set aside 1 c of coconut milk in a small bowl. Sprinkle with gelatin powder and combine well to make a creamy paste. Whisk almost constantly until "paste-like".

Meanwhile, warm, on low, the remaining coconut milk, stirring frequently to make sure it isn't too hot.

Add lime juice, vanilla, and honey to coconut milk and combine well.

Once fully combined, mix in the coconut milk paste. Whisk constantly as it combines with the other coconut milk and is heated through.

NOTE: This does not have to be hot. The heat will help the ingredients combine well, so, once combined, pour mixture into a dish – perhaps a mason jar. Cover and leave in the fridge for at least one hour or up to overnight.

Remove the hardened "yogurt" from the fridge and you'll see that it has taken on a jello-like consistency. If you prefer your yogurt a little runnier, put it into a blender with 1/2 a cup of water to thin it out.

If you like the jello consistency, like I do, sprinkle it with some raisins, cinnamon, honey, and eat immediately!

## NUTRITION VALUE

70 Cal, 8g fat, 1g saturated fat, 13.6g fiber, 22g protein, 1g carbs.

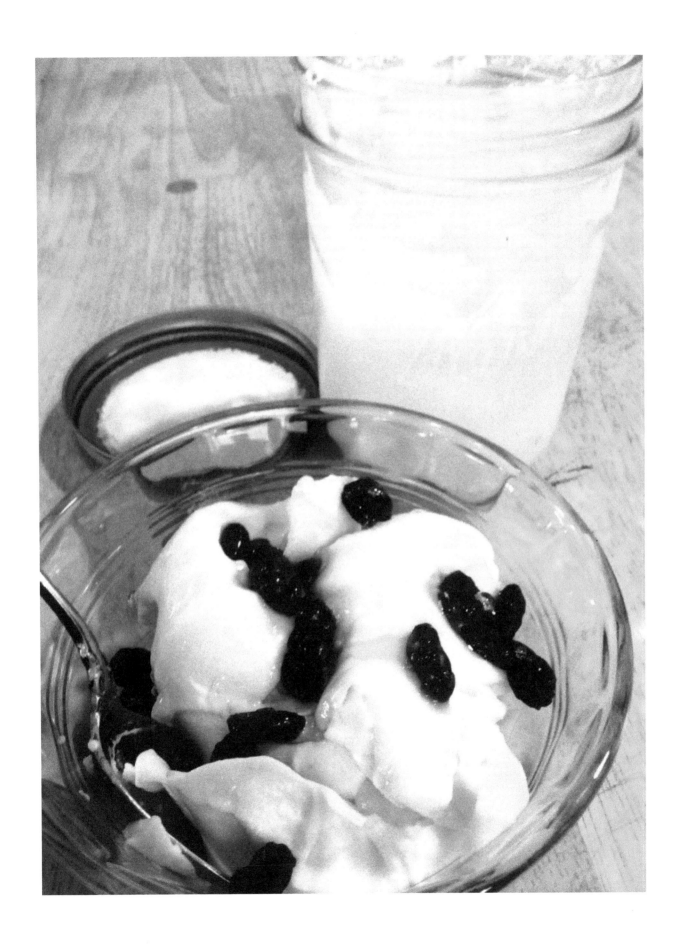

# Lunch

# COCONUT CRUSTED CHICKEN SALAD

As healthy eaters, we are used to having lots of salad. And Chicken Salad is a favorite dish of almost everyone.

MAKES 2 SERVING/ TOTAL TIME 25 MINUTE

## INGREDIENTS

2 tbsp Coconut flour

2 tbsp Unsweetened flaked coconut

2 Chicken fillets

1 Egg (beaten)

2 cups Spring mix salad greens

3 tbsp Apple cider vinegar

1 tsp Honey

3 tbsp olive oil

2 tbsp Coconut oil

Salt and pepper (to taste)

## METHOD

### STEP 1

Create a breading/dredging station with three plates or shallow bowls. Add the coconut flour to one, the egg to the second plate and the flaked coconut to the third. Heat the coconut oil in a skillet over medium-high heat. Dredge each chicken fillet in the coconut flour first, followed by the egg, coating each evenly. Then the flaked coconut. Be sure the fillet is coated well.

Place each fillet into the hot skillet. Cook on each side, about 5 minutes. Until the chicken is golden in color and cooked through.

### STEP 2

Add the apple cider vinegar and honey to a bowl. Whisk to combine. Continue to whisk while drizzling in the olive oil until well combined and becomes creamy. Season with salt and pepper.

Place the spring mix in a mixing bowl. Drizzle the dressing over and toss to coat. Reserve ½ to serving. Plate the spring mix evenly then serve the chicken on top. Serve with additional dressing on the side. Season with salt and pepper, to taste.

| NUTRITION VALUE | 368 Cal, 19g fat, 5g saturated fat, 7g fiber, 21g protein, 14g carbs. |
|---|---|

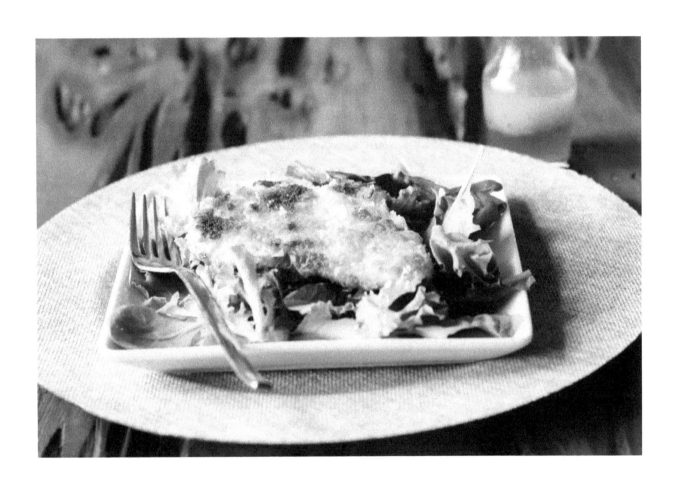

# ZUCCHINI FRITTERS

Spicy and packed with flavor, these zucchini fritters are sure to get you rave reviews in the kitchen.

MAKES 6 SERVING/ TOTAL TIME 20 MINUTE

## INGREDIENTS

2 Zucchini (grated)

1 tsp Sea salt

2 tbsp Coconut flour

4 Scallions (sliced)

1 Egg

1 tsp Cayenne pepper

1 tsp Black pepper

2 tbsp Coconut oil

## METHOD

**STEP 1**

In a medium-sized mixing bowl, stir together the shredded zucchini and sea salt. Set aside for 10 minutes.

After 10 minutes, squeeze the water out of the zucchini and transfer to a clean bowl.

Stir in the coconut flour, egg, scallions, cayenne, and pepper.

**STEP 2**

Add the coconut oil to a medium skillet over medium-high heat.

Once the coconut oil has melted, form six fritters and place them in the skillet. Brown on each side then set aside on a paper-towel lined plate.

Serve immediately. Garnish with additional scallions.

**NUTRITION VALUE**

127 Cal, 11g fat, 2g saturated fat, 2g fiber, 21g protein, 6g carbs.

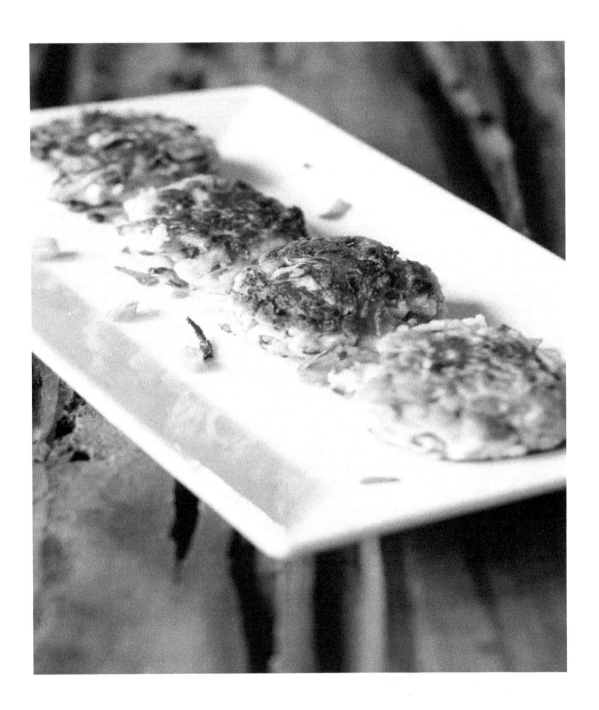

# PORK CABBAGE ROLLS

Pork is a good source of protein that is good for the muscles.

MAKES 4 SERVING/ TOTAL TIME 40 MINUTE

## INGREDIENTS

10 Savory cabbage leaves

1/2 lb. Ground pork

1/2 Onion (minced)

1 Garlic clove (minced)

2 tbsp Coconut aminos

2 tbsp Rice vinegar

1 tbsp Almond meal

1 Egg (beaten)

Chicken broth

## METHOD

### STEP 1

Put the cabbage leaves in a large bowl. Pour boiling water into the bowl, covering the cabbage. Let it set for up to 5 minutes then remove and set aside to cool.

In a medium mixing bowl, add the pork, onion, garlic, ginger, coconut aminos, vinegar, almond meal, and egg. Use your hands to combine the ingredients.

### STEP 2

Form 10 meatball-sized pork balls and set aside.

Place one pork ball onto the center of one cabbage leaf. Fold the sides of the leaf over the ball and tuck them underneath. Repeat with remaining pork balls and cabbage leaves.

Pour enough chicken broth into a stock pot to reach about 1-inch deep. Carefully place the cabbage rolls in the stock pot.

Cover with a tight-fitting lid and turn to medium heat. Cook for 20 to 25 minutes.

Serve immediately.

| NUTRITION VALUE | 179 Cal, 14g fat, 5g saturated fat, 2g fiber, 20g protein, 2g carbs. |
| --- | --- |

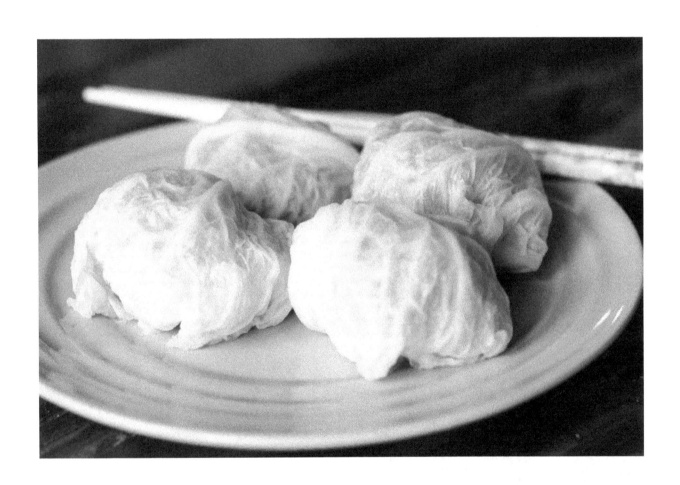

# SAUTÉED KALE

Sautéed kale makes a great paleo side dish or quick lunch.

MAKES 2 SERVING/ TOTAL TIME 10 MINUTE

## INGREDIENTS

4 cups Kale (washed and chopped)

1/4 Onion (diced)

2 Garlic cloves (minced)

1 tbsp olive oil

1 tbsp Red wine vinegar

2 tbsp Almonds (sliced)

Salt (to taste)

## METHOD

**STEP 1**

Heat the olive oil in a skillet over medium heat.
Add the onions and sauté until translucent, about 5 minutes.

**STEP 2**

Add the garlic, kale, almonds, and red wine vinegar.
Cook until the kale is tender, about 5 to 7 minutes.
Season with salt and serve.

**NUTRITION  VALUE**

391 Cal, 18g fat, 2g saturated fat, 11g fiber, 21g protein, 11g carbs.

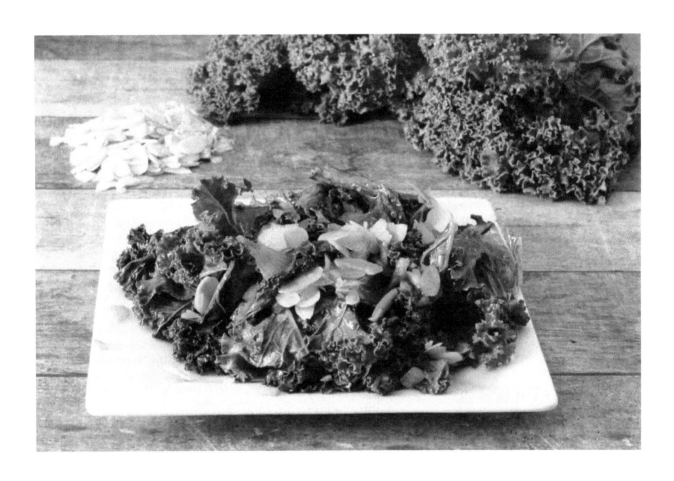

# CHICKEN LETTUCE WRAPS

It's a one-pot meal that can be prepped ahead of time.

MAKES 4 SERVING/ TOTAL TIME 30 MINUTE

## INGREDIENTS

1 lb. Chicken tenders (cut into 1-inch pieces)

1 Onion (diced)

1 Garlic clove (minced)

1 Orange pepper (diced)

5-6 White mushrooms (diced)

3 Celery stalks (diced)

3 Carrots (sliced)

5-6 Brussels sprouts (quartered, stems discarded)

2 tsp Rice vinegar

1 tbsp Coconut aminos

1 tsp Red pepper flake (crushed)

Sea salt and black pepper (to taste)

2 tbsp Coconut oil

1 Head of Iceberg lettuce (leaves separated)

## METHOD

**STEP 1**

Heat the coconut oil in large skillet over medium heat.

Add the onion, celery, pepper, and garlic. Sauté for 2 to 3 minutes, or until the onion is translucent.

Add the chicken. Sauté for 4 to 5 minutes, until beginning to brown, stirring frequently.

Add the mushrooms, carrots, and Brussel sprouts. Sauté for 3 to 4 minutes, stirring frequently.

**STEP 2**

Add the rice vinegar, coconut aminos, ground ginger, and crushed red pepper flake. Stir to coat.

Season with salt and pepper.

Sauté another 2 to 3 minutes or until the chicken is cooked through.

Transfer to a serving platter with the iceberg lettuce.

To eat, spoon about 2 tbsp of the chicken mixture into a lettuce leaf, fold over and eat.

## NUTRITION VALUE

86 Cal, 9g fat, 7g saturated fat, 1g fiber, 20g protein, 5g carbs.

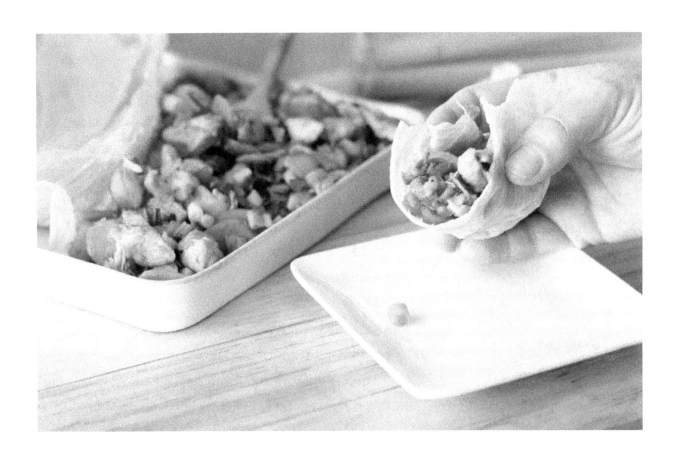

# SWEET POTATO AND CHICKEN CURRY

One of our favorite South Asian cuisine is the Chicken Curry. We made it special by simply adding sweet potatoes.

MAKES 2 SERVING/ TOTAL TIME 20 MINUTE

## INGREDIENTS

1 lb. Chicken breast (cut into 1-inch chunks)

2 tbsp olive oil (divided, coconut oil works as well)

2 Sweet potatoes (large, peeled and cut into 1-inch cubes)

1/2 Onion (diced)

2 Garlic cloves (minced)

1 tbsp Curry powder (use your favorite)

1 tsp Ground ginger

1/2 cup Chicken stock

1 can Coconut milk

Salt (to taste)

Black pepper (to taste)

## METHOD

### STEP 1

Heat 1 tbsp of cooking oil in a large skillet over medium heat. Add the chicken breast chunks and season with salt and pepper. Brown the chicken, about 3-4 minutes per side.

Once the chicken is cooked remove from the pan and set aside. Add the remaining 1 tbsp olive oil to the pan. Add the onions and cook until translucent, about 5-7 minutes.

### STEP 2

Add the garlic, curry powder, and ground ginger then cook for an additional 1-2 minutes, until fragrant.

Add the chicken stock and deglaze the pan, making sure to scrape all the brown bits off the bottom of the pan with a wooden spoon

Add the coconut milk and sweet potatoes. Add the chicken back to the pan.

Bring to a simmer and cover with a tight-fitting lid. Simmer until the sweet potatoes are tender, about 15-20 minutes.

Season with salt and pepper to taste and serve.

| NUTRITION VALUE | 335 Kcal, 14g fat, 8g fiber, 32g protein, 14g carbs. |
|---|---|

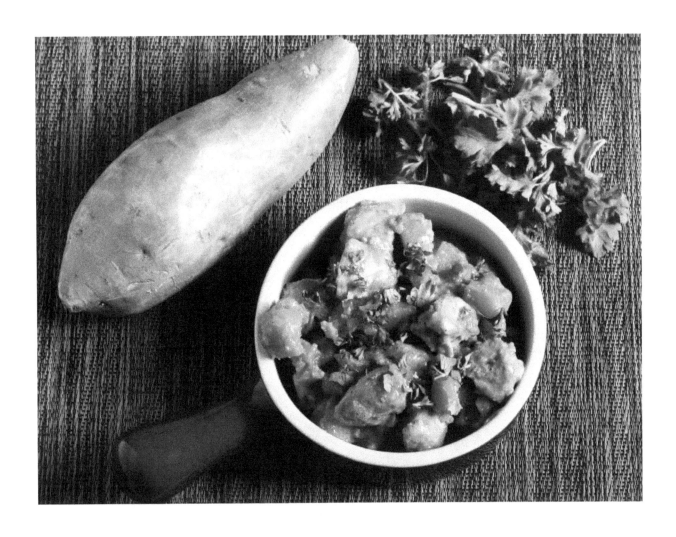

# ITALIAN SAUSAGE AND PEPPERS

This Italian Sausage and Peppers recipe will be a life saver for the nights when you have no idea what to make for dinner. It's incredibly flavorful but also simple to make.

MAKES 4 SERVING/ TOTAL TIME 30 MINUTE

## INGREDIENTS

4 Italian sausages fully cooked, or chicken sausage

2 Bell peppers any color, sliced into strips

1 Red onion sliced

1 tbsp Coconut oil or avocado oil

Fresh parsley optional

Sea salt and black pepper to taste

## METHOD

**STEP 1**

Heat the cooking oil over medium high heat in a large skillet.

Add the sausages. Cook for 4-6 minutes, turning frequently so it browns evenly.

Move the sausages to the sides of the skillet and add the peppers and onions.

**STEP 2**

Sauté the peppers and onions until soft and slightly caramelized.

Transfer the sausages to a cutting board and slice on the diagonal. About 4-5 slices per sausage.

Transfer the peppers and onions to a serving plate. Top with sausage.

Season with sea salt and black pepper, to taste. Garnish with fresh parsley.

| NUTRITION VALUE | 348 Cal, 20g fat, 9g saturated fat, 1g fiber, 21g protein, 2g carbs. |
|---|---|

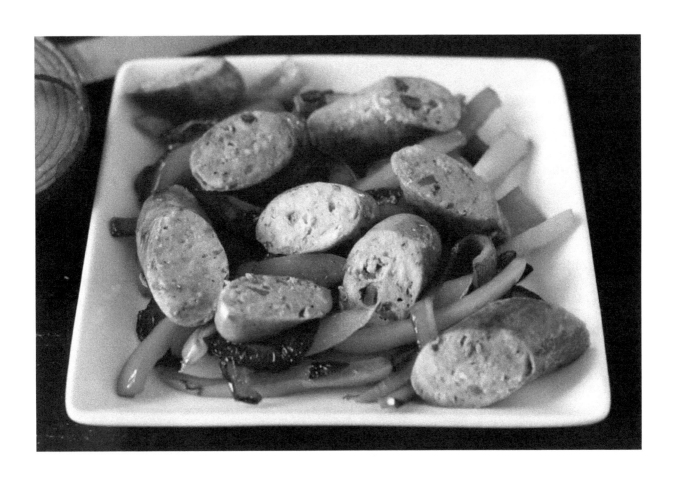

# AVOCADO CHICKEN SALAD

This chicken salad will become a "go-to" paleo lunch for you and your family.

MAKES 4 SERVING/ TOTAL TIME 45 MINUTE

## INGREDIENTS

4 Chicken thighs (boneless and skinless)

1 tsp Chili powder

1 tsp Cumin

1 tsp Sea salt

1 tbsp Avocado oil

3 Avocado

2 Tomatoes (small, diced)

1/2 Red onion (diced)

1 Lime (juice only)

Sea salt and black pepper (to taste)

## METHOD

**STEP 1**

Preheat the oven to 350 degrees. Arrange the chicken thighs in a glass baking dish.

Season with chili powder, cumin and sea salt.

Drizzle with oil. Add chicken to preheated oven and cook for 20-30 minutes or until chicken is cooked through and no longer pink. Remove chicken and shred with 2 forks. Set aside to cool.

**STEP 2**

In a mixing bowl, add the avocado. Use the back of a fork to mash it slightly. You want some bits of avocado and some creamy.

Add the tomato, onion, and lime juice.

Add the chicken. Stir to combine.

Season with sea salt and black pepper. Serve immediately.

Store in an airtight container with a piece of plastic wrap pressed directly on top of the salad in order to prevent avocado browning.

**NUTRITION VALUE**

530 Cal, 20g fat, 11g saturated fat, 7g fiber, 21g protein, 14g carbs.

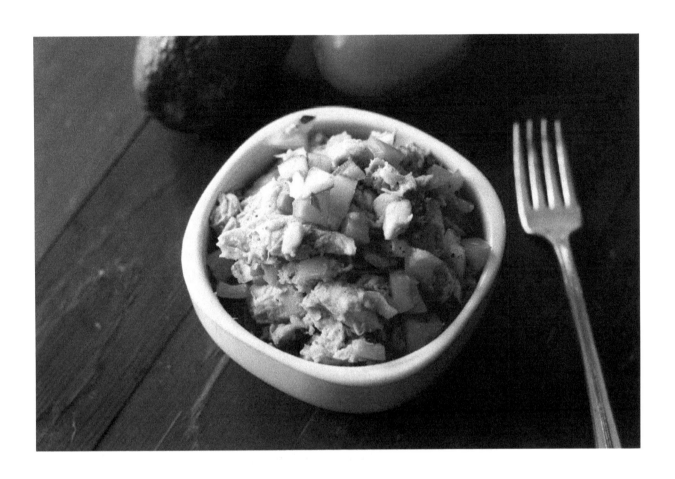

# PALEO SLOPPY JOES

This is the perfect quick weeknight meal. Serve it with a side of steamed vegetables or a salad and you have the perfect meal.

MAKES 4 SERVING/ TOTAL TIME 20 MINUTE

## INGREDIENTS

1 lb. Ground beef (or turkey)

1 Bell pepper (diced)

1 Onion (diced)

3 Celery stalks (diced)

1 Garlic clove (minced)

1 tsp Cumin

1 tsp Chili powder

2 cups Tomato sauce

1/4 tsp Cayenne pepper (optional)

1/4 tsp Red pepper flake (optional)

Sea salt (to taste)

Fresh cracked black pepper (to taste)

Coconut oil

## METHOD

### STEP 1

Heat the coconut oil over medium high heat in a large skillet.

Add the onion, pepper, and celery and sauté for 4-5 minutes, or until the vegetables are soft.

Add the garlic, sauté for 2-3 minutes.

Add the ground beef and cook until browned and cooked through.

### STEP 2

Add the tomato sauce and spices. Stir to combine.

Scrape any bits off the bottom of the skillet.

Cook on medium heat until the sauce thicken a bit, about 10 minutes.

Serve hot with a side of steamed vegetables.

## NUTRITION VALUE

330 Cal, 20g fat, 8g saturated fat, 2g fiber, 31g protein, 11g carbs.

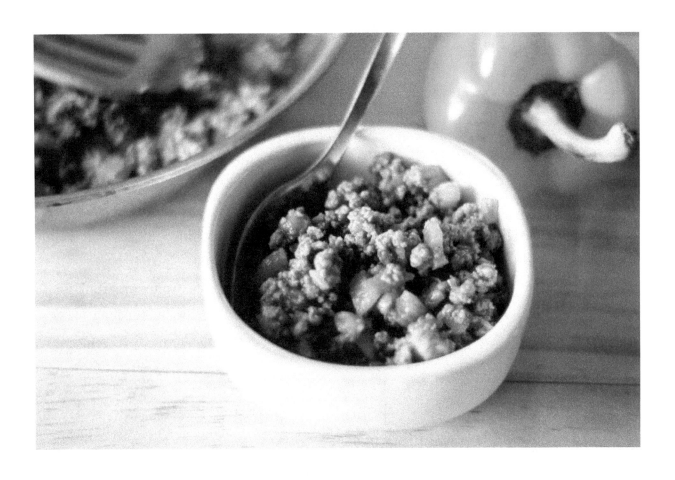

# PESTO STUFFED SARDINES

Sardines are a nutrient dense food packed full of vitamins, minerals and healthy fats.

MAKES 1 SERVING/ TOTAL TIME 20 MINUTE

## INGREDIENTS

Pesto

2 cups Fresh spinach (packed)

1 Garlic clove

1/4 cup Almonds

2 tbsp olive oil

Salt (to taste)

Sardines

6 Fresh sardines (cleaned)

2 tbsp Coconut oil (melted)

Salt (to taste)

Black pepper (to taste)

## METHOD

### STEP 1

Preheat the broiler. Place the top shelf about 6 inches from the broiler in your oven.

Combine all the ingredients for the pesto in a food processor. Blend until a paste forms. Set aside.

Rinse the sardines and pat dry with a paper towel.

Place the sardines on a foil lined baking sheet.

Stuff each sardine with 1 tbsp of the pesto.

### STEP 2

Brush both sides of the sardine with coconut oil and season with salt and pepper.

Place the sardine sunder the broiler and cook for 4 minutes on each side, until cooked through.

Remove from the oven and serve.

| NUTRITION VALUE | 242 Cal, 20g fat, 8g saturated fat, 5g fiber, 21g protein, 7g carbs. |
| --- | --- |

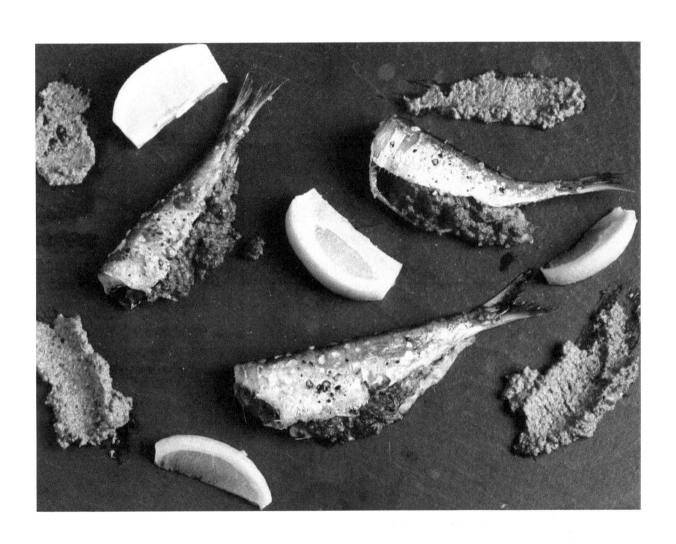

# BACON JALAPEÑO MASHED SWEET POTATOES

These potatoes are definitely a break from the ordinary. They are the perfect combination of sweet and spicy.

MAKES 4 SERVING/ TOTAL TIME 1 HOUR

## INGREDIENTS

4 Sweet potatoes

2 Jalapeños diced

4 strips bacon cooked until crispy and chopped

1/2 cup Coconut cream

Sea salt and black pepper to taste

## METHOD

### STEP 1

Preheat the oven to 400 degrees F. Place the sweet potatoes on a baking sheet and add to preheated oven. Cook for 40-45 minutes or until the potatoes are fork tender. (a fork goes in easily)

Remove the sweet potatoes from the oven and set aside to rest. About 5-6 minutes.

Once the potatoes have cooled enough to handle, cut them in half and scoop the inside into a bowl. Add the coconut cream and jalapeno. Stir well to combine. If you want creamier potatoes, use an immersion blender or hand mixer. Fold in half the bacon.

### STEP 2

Transfer the potatoes to a serving bowl and garnish the top with bacon. Season with sea salt and black pepper.

Serve immediately.

## NUTRITION VALUE

415 Cal, 20g fat, 7g saturated fat, 4g fiber, 22g protein, 14g carbs.

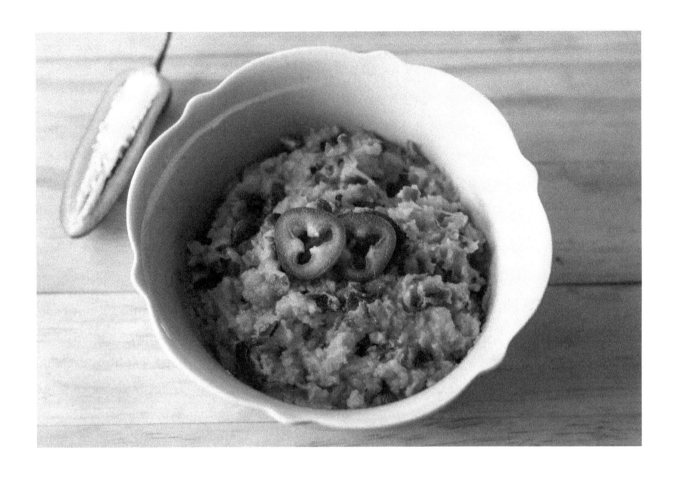

# CURRY CAULIFLOWER RICE

One of the hardest things for anyone new to Paleo to give up is a side of rice with their curry.

MAKES 2 SERVING/ TOTAL TIME 15 MINUTE

## INGREDIENTS

1 head Cauliflower

1 tbsp olive oil

1/4 tsp Curry powder

1/4 tsp Turmeric

1/8 tsp Ginger ground

Salt to taste

Fresh parsley chopped, to garnish

## METHOD

### STEP 1

Cut the cauliflower into florets, making sure to get a little stem as possible. If you accidentally cut large stems make sure to trim them.

Put the cauliflower in a food processor and pulse until it becomes a rice consistency.

### STEP 2

Heat the olive oil in a skillet over medium heat. Add the cauliflower rice and sauté for 4-5 minutes, until soft. While the cauliflower rice is cooking mix together the spices in a small bowl. Stir into the cauliflower making sure to coat evenly. Cook for 1-2 minutes until fragrant. Season with salt and remove from the heat.

Garnish with fresh parsley and serve.

**NUTRITION VALUE**

70 Cal, 8g fat, 1g saturated fat, 13.6g fiber, 22g protein, 1g carbs.

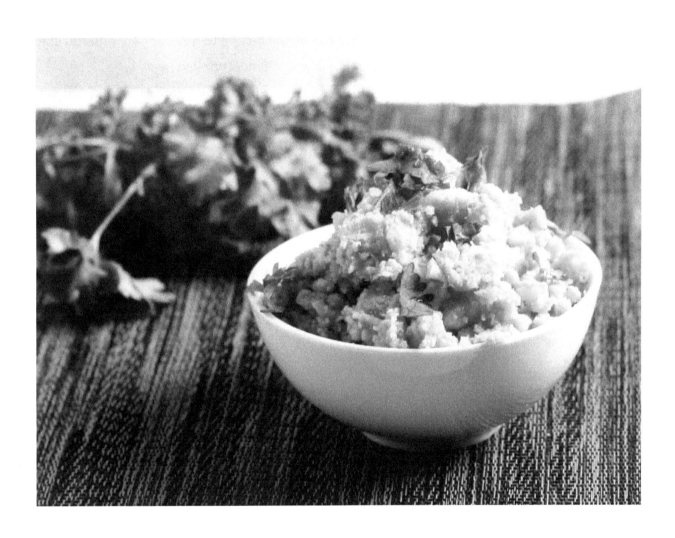

# CHICKEN "TACO" BAR

This taco bar is a fun way to make your dinner a social experience.

MAKES 6 SERVING/ TOTAL TIME 20 MINUTE

## INGREDIENTS

6 Chicken breasts and

1/2 tsp Ground cumin

1/2 tsp Chili powder

1/8 tsp Cayenne pepper optional

1/2 tsp Garlic powder

1/4 tsp Onion powder

1/4 tsp Ground mustard

1/2 tsp Dried oregano

1/2 tsp Sea salt

1/2 cup Chicken broth

12-16 Romaine leaves

2 Tomatoes diced

1/2 cup Carrot shredded

1/2 cup Cabbage shredded

4-6 slices bacon cooked crispy

1-2 Avocados diced

1 cup Broccoli shredded or diced

## METHOD

### STEP 1

Add the cooked chicken to a sauce pan. Add the chicken broth. Turn on to medium low heat.

Add the cumin, chili powder, garlic powder, cayenne, onion powder, ground mustard, and oregano. Stir to combine.

### STEP 2

Bring the chicken mixture to a simmer, then turn down to low. Cook until the broth has thickened slightly and chicken is heated through.

Add the topping items to individual serving bowl.

Stack the romaine lettuce leaves on a plate for serving.

**NUTRITION VALUE**

331 Kcal, 20g fat,
5g fiber, 22g protein, 13g carbs.

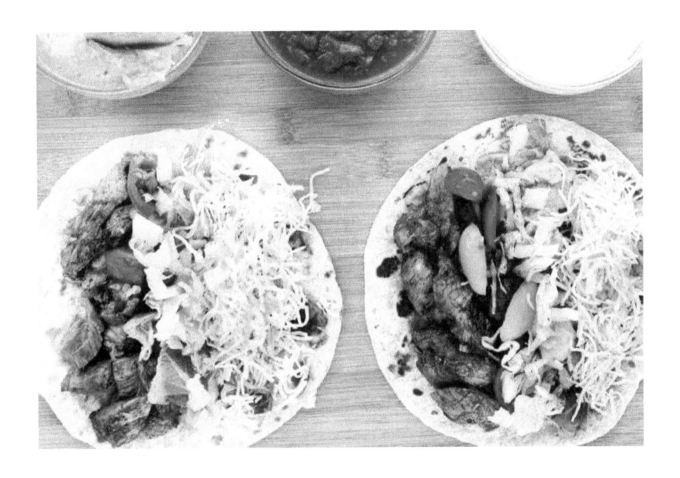

# CREAMY ONE-POT CHICKEN & VEGETABLES

This colorful dish incorporates lots of **veggies** to make sure that your body stays nourished with plenty of vitamins and minerals.

MAKES 4 SERVING/ TOTAL TIME 20 MINUTE

## INGREDIENTS

2-3 Boneless skinless chicken breasts

1/2 c Bacon bits (chopped, about 4 strips of bacon)

1 Red pepper (diced)

1 Yellow pepper (diced)

2 c Fresh kale (washed and torn, stems removed)

2 c Fresh mushrooms (sliced)

1/2 c Onions (diced)

3 tbsp garlic (minced)

1 can Coconut milk (about 2 c)

1/2 tbsp Apple cider vinegar

1 tbsp Arrowroot powder

Salt and pepper (to taste)

Chopped fresh parsley (for garnish)

Crushed red peppers (for garnish)

## METHOD

### STEP 1

Cook bacon in pan and set aside. Chop when cool.

Using bacon fat, sauté onions and garlic for about 3 minutes.

Add in chicken, peppers, and mushrooms. Cook on medium until chicken is no longer pink and vegetables are steamed.

Add vinegar and all but 1/4 cup of the coconut milk.

### STEP 2

Put remaining coconut milk in mason jar with arrowroot powder and shake well with lid on to combine. Pour into chicken skillet.

Add in fresh kale and bring entire pot to light boil for about 5 minutes more.

Serve hot and garnish with parsley and crushed red pepper.

## NUTRITION VALUE

260 Cal, 13g fat, 4g saturated fat, 3g fiber, 21g protein, 14g carbs.

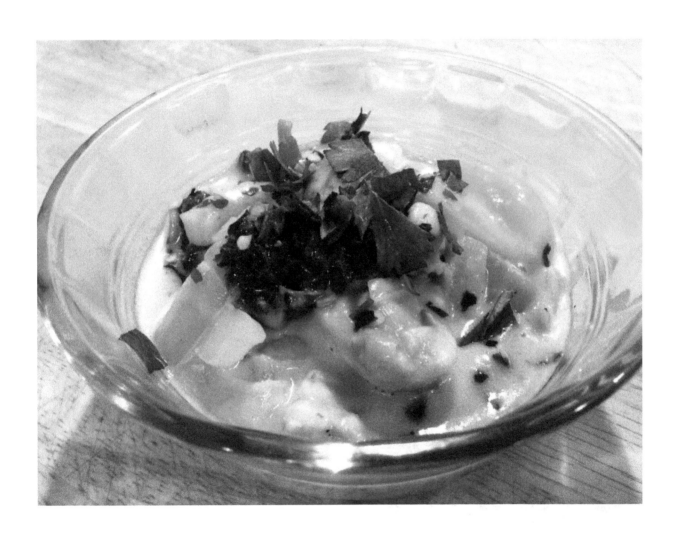

# TWICE BAKED SWEET POTATO

This paleo diet cuisine is highly respected and recognized for its attributes.

## INGREDIENTS

2 Sweet potatoes

Coconut oil

Sea salt

1 c Chicken (shredded)

1/3 c Fresh green onions (diced)

Avocado (sliced, optional garnish)

Hot sauce (optional garnish)

Fried egg (optional garnish)

## METHOD

### STEP 1

Preheat oven to 350 degrees.

Poke sweet potatoes all over with a knife and use hands to slather some coconut oil onto the skins. Lightly sprinkle with sea salt and cook for 1 hour at 350 degrees.

### STEP 2

Once potatoes are done, cut open, and stuff with shredded chicken. Place back into the oven for 15 minutes or until middle is warmed through. Garnish with fresh chopped green onion, sliced avocado, hot sauce, and/or a fried egg.

**NUTRITION VALUE**

243 Cal, 9g fat, 3g saturated fat, 1g fiber, 36g protein, 3g carbs.

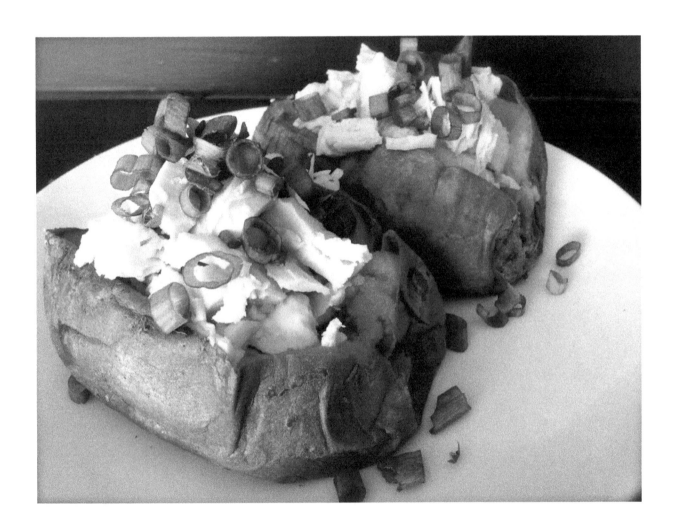

# Dinner

# CRISPY CAULIFLOWER CAKES

Cauliflower has many health benefits such as vitamin C, vitamin K, folate, pantothenic acid, and vitamin B6.

MAKES 6 SERVING/ TOTAL TIME 30 MINUTE

## INGREDIENTS

1 head Cauliflower

1 tbsp Ghee (or Coconut oil, melted)

2 tsp Garlic powder

2 tbsp chives (chopped)

3 tbsp Coconut flour

2 Eggs (beaten)

1 tsp Salt

2-4 tbsp Coconut oil (for frying)

## METHOD

### STEP 1

Cut the cauliflower into florets. Place the florets in a food processor and pulse until they become a rice like texture. Transfer the riced cauliflower to a large microwave-safe mixing bowl and microwave on high for 2 to 3 minutes, until cooked through.

Remove the bowl from the microwave and set aside to cool for about 5 minutes. Add the melted ghee (or coconut oil), chopped chives, garlic powder, coconut flour, eggs, and salt to the mixing bowl. Mix until all the ingredients are well combined.

Use your hands to form the mixture into 6 to 8 patties. Set aside.

### STEP 2

Heat the coconut oil in a skillet over medium heat. Fry the patties in the coconut oil until browned, about 2 to 3 minutes per side. Remove the patties from the oil and place on a paper towel lined plate to remove any excess oil.

## NUTRITION VALUE

86 Cal, 8.7g fat, 7g saturated fat, 3g fiber, 2g protein, 6g carbs.

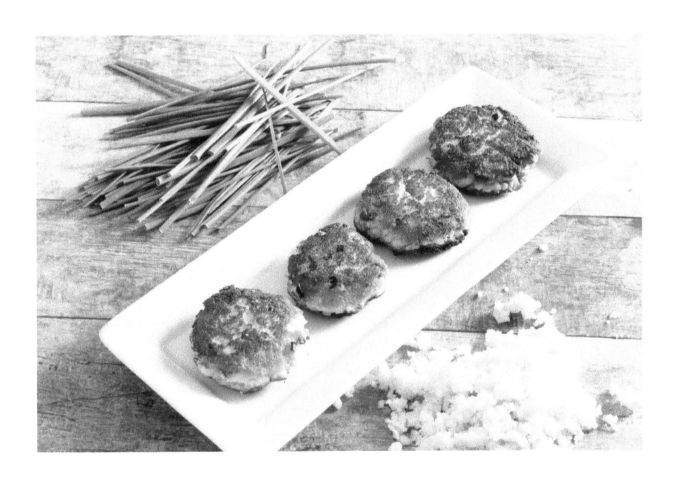

# ROASTED BEETROOT HUMMUS

Roasted beets are a year-round, must-eat staple in the house. Beets are filled with good-for-you nutrients and bring out their natural sweetness when roasted.

MAKES 2 SERVING/ TOTAL TIME 45 MINUTE

## INGREDIENTS

2 Beets (peeled and cut into quarters)

1/4 cup Olive oil (plus more for drizzling)

1 Zucchini (peeled and cut into chunks)

1/4 cup Tahini

1/2 Lemon (juiced)

Salt (to taste)

5-6 Carrots (peeled and cut into sticks)

## METHOD

**STEP 1**

Preheat the oven to 400 degrees F.

Place the beet quarters on a baking sheet. Drizzle with a little olive oil and season with salt. Place in the oven and bake for 20 to 30 minutes, until the beets are fork tender. Remove from the oven and set aside to cool for about 10 minutes.

**STEP 2**

In a food processor combine the roasted beets, chopped zucchini, tahini, lemon juice, and olive oil. Blend until smooth. Season with salt to taste.
Serve with carrot sticks and enjoy!

**NUTRITION VALUE**

368 Cal, 19g fat, 5g saturated fat, 7g fiber, 21g protein, 14g carbs.

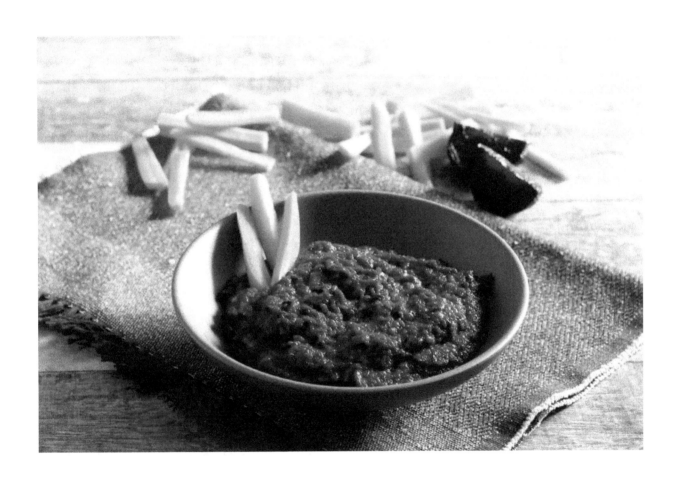

# BEEF MASAMAN CURRY

There are few things more comforting than a warm bowl of delicious curry.

MAKES 3 SERVING/ TOTAL TIME 40 MINUTE

## INGREDIENTS

1 1/2 lbs. Skirt Steak (cut into 1 1/2-inch cubes)

1 tbsp Coconut oil

1/2 Onion (finely chopped)

3 tbsp Masaman curry paste

1 can Coconut milk

2 cups Spinach

2 tbsp Cilantro (chopped)

1 head Cauliflower

Salt (to taste)

## METHOD

### STEP 1

Cut the cauliflower into florets. Place the florets in a food processor and pulse until it takes on a rice like texture. Transfer to a microwave bowl and microwave on high for 3 to 4 minutes, until cooked through. Remove from the microwave and set aside.

Heat the coconut oil in a skillet over medium heat. Add the beef and brown, about 2 to 3 minutes per side. Remove from the pan and set aside.

Add the onion to the pan and sauté until translucent, about 5 to 7 minutes.

### STEP 2

Add the curry paste to the pan and sauté for 1 to 2 minutes, until fragrant.

Stir in the coconut milk. Add the beef back to the pan. Add the spinach. Cover and reduce heat to a simmer. Simmer for 20 minutes. Add the fresh cilantro and season with salt to taste.

Serve the masaman curry over the cauliflower rice and enjoy!

| NUTRITION VALUE | 335 Kcal, 14g fat, 8g fiber, 32g protein, 14g carbs. |
|---|---|

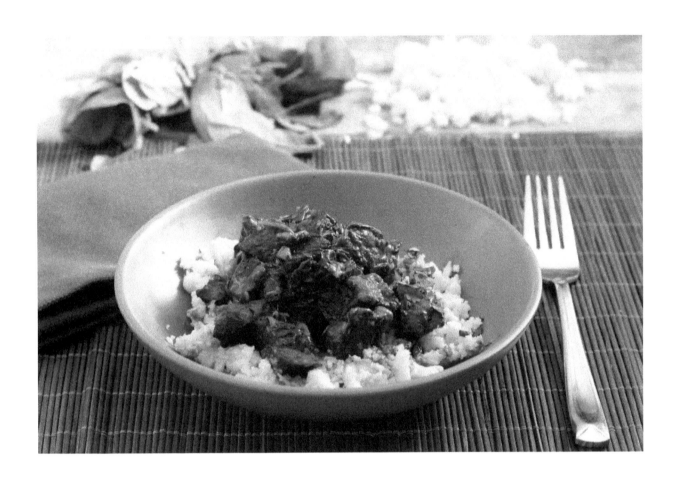

# SWEET POTATO SOUP WITH BACON

Full of Thanksgiving flavors, this sweet potato soup with bacon is comfort in a bowl–plus everything is better with bacon.

MAKES 6 SERVING/ TOTAL TIME 7 HOUR

## INGREDIENTS

2 lbs. Sweet potatoes (peeled and roughly chopped)

2 cups Chicken stock

1 tbsp Ground cinnamon

1 tbsp Ground nutmeg

1 tsp Ground ginger

1/2 cup Coconut milk

4 slices bacon (cooked crisply and diced)

## METHOD

**STEP 1**

Add the sweet potatoes, chicken stock, cinnamon, nutmeg, and ginger to the slow cooker.

Cook on low for 6 hours.

**STEP 2**

Add the coconut milk and use your immersion blender to blend until creamy.

Serve hot topped with bacon.

| NUTRITION VALUE | 169 Cal, 4g fat, 3g saturated fat, 5g fiber, 20g protein, 14g carbs. |
|---|---|

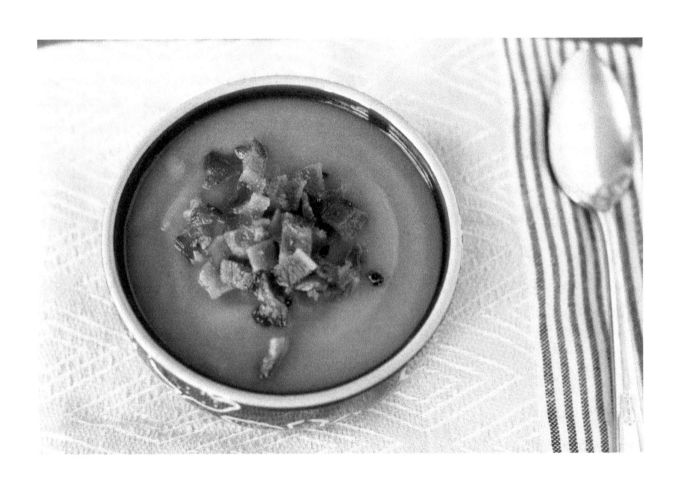

# SLOW COOKER PULLED PORK

Pulled pork is one of those wonderful and delicious treats that reminds us of warm weather, picnics and hanging out with friends.

MAKES 4 SERVING/ TOTAL TIME 30 MINUTE

## INGREDIENTS

2 tbsp Ghee

24 oz Tomatoes

6 oz Tomato paste

1/3 cup Apple cider vinegar

1/4 cup Honey

1/3 cup Blackstrap molasses

2 tbsp Chipotle chili powder

1 tbsp Onion powder

1 tbsp Garlic powder

2 tbsp Ground mustard

1 tsp Salt

3-4 lb. Pork shoulder

1 yellow onion

1/2 cup Apple cider vinegar

1/4 cup Honey

1/3 cup olive oil

1/4 tsp Garlic powder

1/2 tsp Celery seed

## METHOD

### STEP 1

BBQ Sauce: Add the ghee to a pot over medium heat. Stir until melted. Add the remaining ingredients to the pot. Bring the mixture to a simmer. Simmer for 15 minutes, stirring occasionally to prevent burning. Remove from the burner and set aside to cool.

### STEP 2

Pulled Pork: Pour half the BBQ sauce in the bottom of the slow cooker. Sprinkle the sliced onion on top of the sauce. Place the pork shoulder on top of the onions. Season with salt. Pour the remaining BBQ sauce over the pork. Secure the lid and cook for 8 hours on low. Once the pork is done cooking, use a fork to shred the meat.

### STEP 3

Coleslaw: In a large bowl whisk together the apple cider vinegar, honey, olive oil, salt, garlic powder, and celery seed. Mix in the coleslaw vegetables.

Serve the pulled pork with the coleslaw and enjoy!

**NUTRITION VALUE**

415 Cal, 20g fat, 7g saturated fat, 4g fiber, 22g protein, 14g carbs.

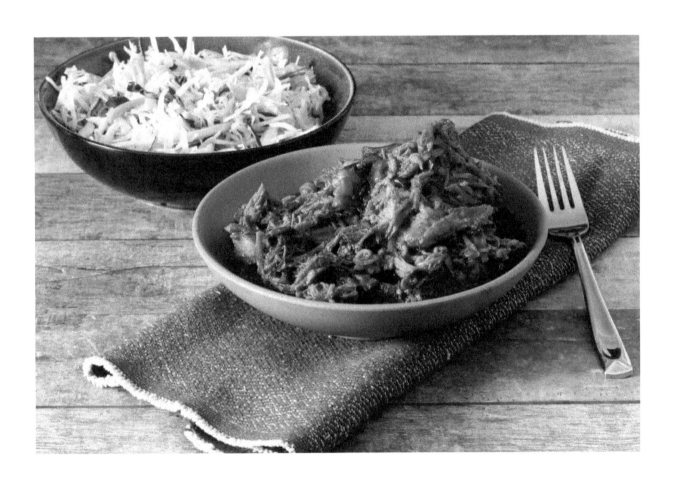

# LEMON AND THYME ROASTED CHICKEN BREAST

Chicken meat is a very good source of the nutrient for the muscles – protein.

MAKES 2 SERVING/ TOTAL TIME 35 MINUTE

## INGREDIENTS

2 Boneless and skinless chicken breasts

1 Lemon

6-7 Sprigs of thyme (stems discarded)

1 tbsp olive oil (plus more for drizzling)

Salt and pepper (to taste)

## METHOD

**STEP 1**

Place the chicken in a sealable container or zip top bag. Squeeze the lemon over the chicken.

Add the thyme and olive oil. Toss to coat and season with salt. Set aside in the refrigerator for at least 30 minutes up to 8 hours.

**STEP 2**

Preheat the oven to 350 degrees F.

Place the chicken in a baking dish and drizzle with additional olive oil.

Bake in preheated oven for 30 minutes or until chicken is cooked.

Pepper to taste.

## NUTRITION VALUE

530 Cal, 20g fat, 11g saturated fat, 7g fiber, 21g protein, 14g carbs.

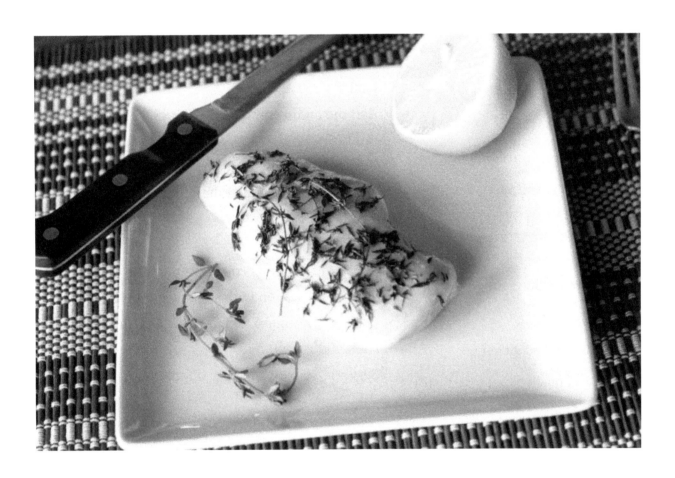

# CASHEW CHICKEN

This recipe combines so many flavors that are all brought together with the cashews.

MAKES 4 SERVING/ TOTAL TIME 30 MINUTE

## INGREDIENTS

2 Boneless and skinless chicken breasts (cut into 1 chunks)

1 Red bell pepper (cut into strips)

1 Onion (cut into strips)

1 Garlic cloves (minced)

1/2 cup Raw cashews

2 tbsp Coconut oil

2 tbsp Honey

1 tbsp Coconut aminos

1 tbsp Rice vinegar

1 tsp Fresh grated ginger

Sea salt and black pepper (to taste)

3 Scallions (sliced)

## METHOD

### STEP 1

Pour the coconut oil onto a large skillet over medium heat.

Add the onion and red pepper and cook for a few minutes.

Toss in the chicken and cook for 4 to 5 minutes.

Mix in the garlic and cashews. Cook for another 2 to 3 minutes.

### STEP 2

Stir in the honey, coconut aminos, rice vinegar, grated ginger and season with salt and pepper.

Cook for another 4 to 5 minutes or until the chicken is cooked through.

Serve and garnish with scallions.

| NUTRITION VALUE | 91 Cal, 7g fat, 7g saturated fat, 1g fiber, 11.3g protein, 5g carbs. |
|---|---|

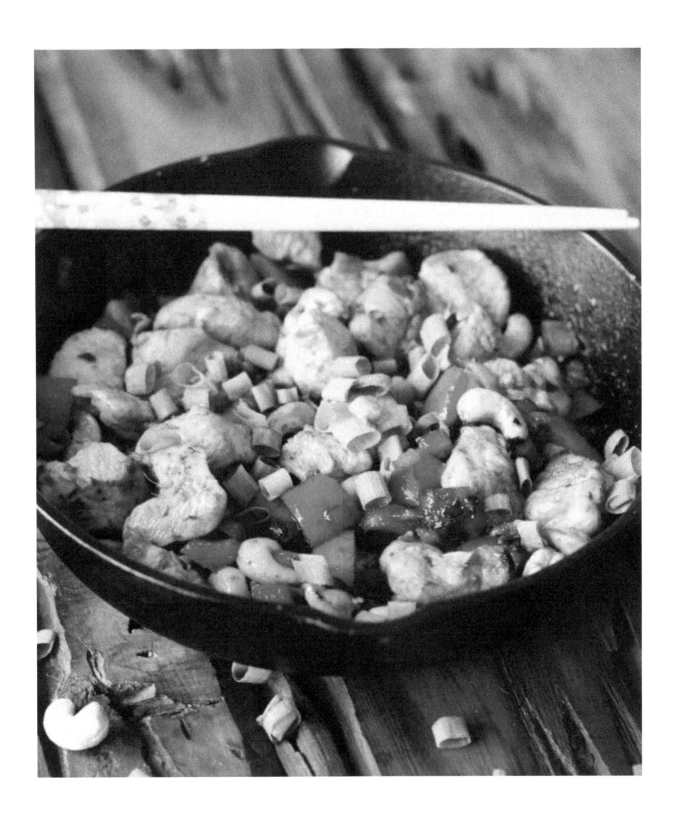

# ALMOND PESTO CRUSTED COD

Cod is a good source of omega 3 and fatty acids that helps in improving the functioning of the human heart muscles, thereby keeping a person safe from the risk of an ischemic stroke.

MAKES 1 SERVING/ TOTAL TIME 15 MINUTE

## INGREDIENTS

For Pesto

2 cups Arugula

3 tbsp Almonds (sliced)

1/2 Lemon (juiced)

1/4 cup olive oil

Salt (to taste)

For Fish

2 tbsp Almonds (ground)

2 tbsp Pesto

5 oz Cod

Salt (to taste)

For Noodles

1 tbsp olive oil

1 Zucchini (or 1/2 large Zucchini, spiralized or julienned)

1/4 cup Pesto

Salt (to taste)

1/4 cup Cherry tomatoes (halved

## METHOD

Preheat oven to 350 degrees F.

Add the 2 tbsp of almonds to a good processor and grind. Set aside. Add the ingredients for the pesto to a food processor. Blend on high until smooth. Set aside. In a small bowl mix together the 2 tbsp almond meal and 2 tbsp of the pesto. Pat the piece of cod dry with a paper towel. Place the fish on a baking sheet. Season the fish with salt. Take the pesto and ground almonds and spoon it on top of the fish, pressing it down slightly to form a crust.

Place the fish in the oven and bake for 8-10 minutes. While the fish is cooking heat the olive oil over medium heat in a skillet. Add the zucchini noodles and ¼ cup pesto (or the rest of the pesto if it is almost gone). Sauté until the noodles are tender, about 3-4 minutes. Season with salt to taste.

Spoon the noodles onto a plate.

When the fish is done remove from the oven. Place the fish over the noodles, garnish with cherry tomatoes and serve.

## NUTRITION VALUE

900 Cal, 20g fat,
20g fiber, 50g protein, 14g carbs.

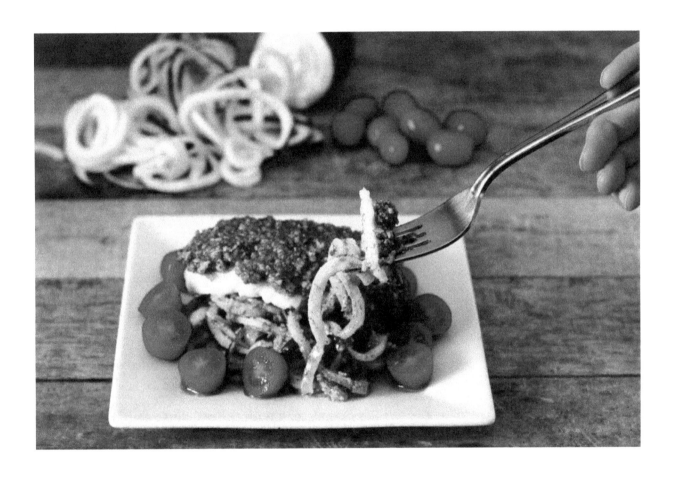

# CLASSIC STEAK AND EGGS

Steak and eggs diet is really mainstream. It is probably a fact that nobody doesn't love steak and eggs.

MAKES 4 SERVING/ TOTAL TIME 25 MINUTE

## INGREDIENTS

4 Steaks sirloin or T-bone, room temperature

3 tsp Cracked peppercorns fresh

1 tsp Sea salt

1 tsp Garlic powder

1 tsp Red pepper flakes

Cooking oil such as olive or coconut

6 Eggs

4 slices Tomato

## METHOD

### STEP 1

Grease the grill pan or grill grates with the cooking oil using a heat proof basting brush.

Heat the grill pan or outdoor grill to medium heat.

Add the peppercorn, salt, garlic powder, and pepper flakes in a bowl and combine.

Rub the spice mixture on the steak on all sides.

Add the steaks and grill for 5-7 minutes (for medium rare) or until the steak is cooked to the desired temperature.

### STEP 2

Set aside to rest.

Heat coconut oil in a nonstick skillet over medium high heat.

Crack one egg at a time and cook until desired doneness.

Serve the steak with the egg and a tomato slice. Season with salt and pepper.

| NUTRITION VALUE | 346 Cal, 13g fat, 3g saturated fat, 2g fiber, 47g protein, 9g carbs. |
|---|---|

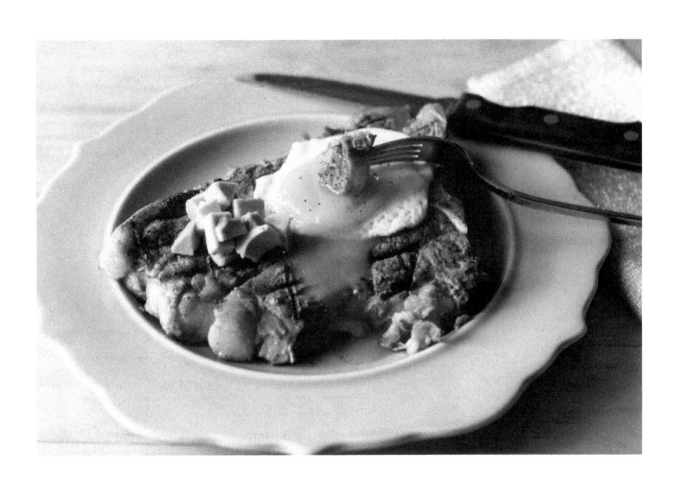

# SLOW COOKER CARNE ASADA

This is the perfect Mexican inspired paleo dinner.

MAKES 4 SERVING/ TOTAL TIME 30 MINUTE

## INGREDIENTS

2 lbs. Sirloin steaks boneless

2 Onions diced

3 Garlic cloves minced

1 Jalapeno seeded and diced

1 Red bell pepper diced

3 Tomatoes roughly chopped

1 4 oz Green chiles diced

1/3 cup Beef broth

2 tbsp Chili powder

1 tbsp Cumin

1/4 tsp Cayenne

1/4 tsp Red pepper flake

Sea salt and black pepper to taste

8-10 Romaine leaves

## METHOD

**STEP 1**

Season the steak with salt and pepper.

Add ½ the onion to the bottom of the slow cooker.

Place the steak on top of the onion.

Add the remaining onion, red bell pepper, jalapeno, tomato, green chiles, chili powder, cumin, cayenne, and red pepper flake.

Gently stir to combine.

**STEP 2**

Add the beef broth.

Set the slow cooker for 6-7 hour on low.

About 30-45 minutes before the slow cooker is done.

Remove the steak, shred with two forks and return to the slow cooker for remainder of cook time.

Serve in a romaine lettuce leaf with a side or topping of guacamole.

Other optional toppings are, homemade salsa, shredded cabbage, fresh cilantro, fresh tomatoes, paleo friendly hot sauce, and lime wedges.

**NUTRITION VALUE**

470 Kcal, 20g fat, 3g fiber, 21g protein, 14g carbs.

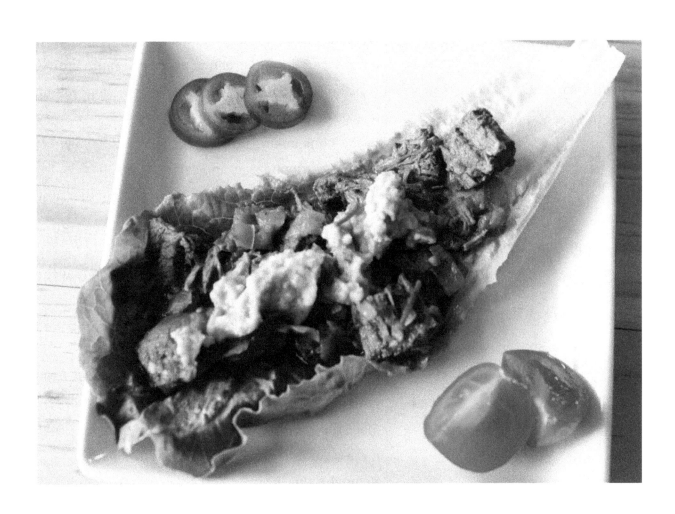

# MINI PALEO MEATLOAVES

These mini paleo meatloaves are sure to be a hit at your family dinner table.

MAKES 3 SERVING/ TOTAL TIME 45 MINUTE

## INGREDIENTS

1 lb. Turkey

1 tbsp olive oil

1/4 Onion minced

1/4 cup Carrots diced fine

1/4 cup Green pepper diced fine

1/4 tsp Marjoram

1/4 tsp Thyme

1 Egg

1/4 tsp Salt

1/4 tsp Black pepper

1/4 cup Paleo Ketchup

6 oz Tomato paste

1/4 cup Honey

1/2 cup White wine vinegar

1/4 cup Water

3/4 tsp Salt

1/8 tsp Onion powder

1/8 tsp Garlic powder

## METHOD

### STEP 1

Preheat oven to 350 degrees F.

Heat the olive oil in a skillet over medium heat. Add the onions, carrots and green peppers and sauté until translucent, about 3-5 minutes. Pour the ingredients in a large mixing bowl.

In the same mixing bowl add the ground turkey, marjoram, thyme, egg, and salt and pepper.

Use your hands to mix the ingredients together, until well combined.

### STEP 2

Form the meat mixture into 8-10 individual loaves and place them on a foil lined baking sheet.

In another bowl whisk together the ingredients for the paleo ketchup.

Spread some of the paleo ketchup on top of each of the individual meatloaves.

Place the meatloaves in the oven and bake for 20-25 minutes, until cooked all the way through.

Remove from the oven and serve warm

## NUTRITION VALUE

255 Cal, 17g fat, 2g saturated fat, 6g fiber, 20g protein, 14g carbs.

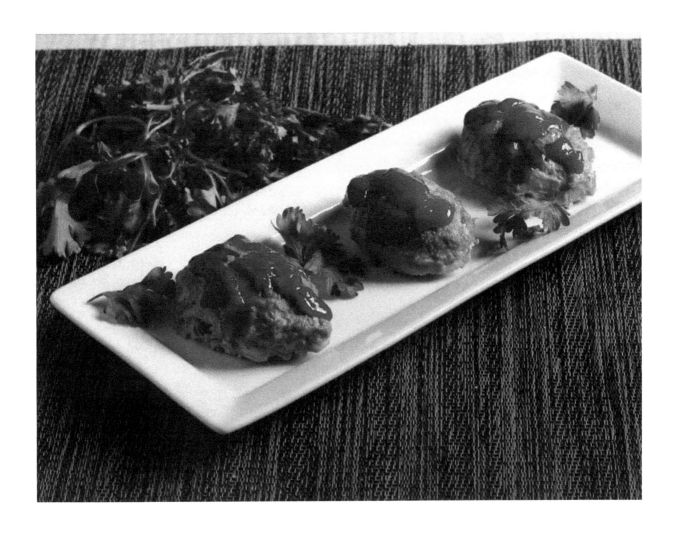

# PALEO VENISON BURGERS

Burger will always be everybody's favorite. Aside from the fact that they are delicious and tasty, burgers are undeniably satisfying.

MAKES 1 SERVING/ TOTAL TIME 10 MINUTE

## INGREDIENTS

1 lb. Ground venison meat

1 tbsp Onion powder

1 tbsp Garlic powder

1/2 c Parsley (fresh chopped)

Sea salt and pepper (to taste)

1 c Sliced onions

1 tbsp Balsamic vinegar

1 tbsp Bacon fat (or other cooking fat)

1 Egg (optional)

## METHOD

In a large mixing bowl, combine ground venison with garlic powder, onion powder, salt, pepper, and chopped parsley.

Use your hands to combine everything together and form the mixture into 4-5 patties. Please note that game meat is much less fatty than other meats, so it won't stick quite the same as other meat does. If you're worried that the patties won't stay firm while cooking, feel free to add one whisked egg to the mix before forming into patties.

Once patties are ready, set them aside and bring a large pan to high heat and melt your cooking fat. As mentioned, these suckers are quite lean, so don't skimp on the cooking fat. Bacon grease adds a really nice flavor to these burgers, in my opinion.

Once the pan is nice and hot, add the burgers, cover them, and cook them for about 3-4 minutes on each side.

Once everything is cooked through, remove the burgers from the pan and turn off the heat. Add 1 tbsp of balsamic vinegar to the onions left in the pan and deglaze the pan and drippings with the vinegar. Combine well with the onions.

Spoon caramelized onions and "gravy" over the top of the burgers and serve hot with fresh steamed veggies like asparagus!

| NUTRITION VALUE | 393 Cal, 20g fat, 9g saturated fat, 12g fiber, 31g protein, 14g carbs. |
|---|---|

76

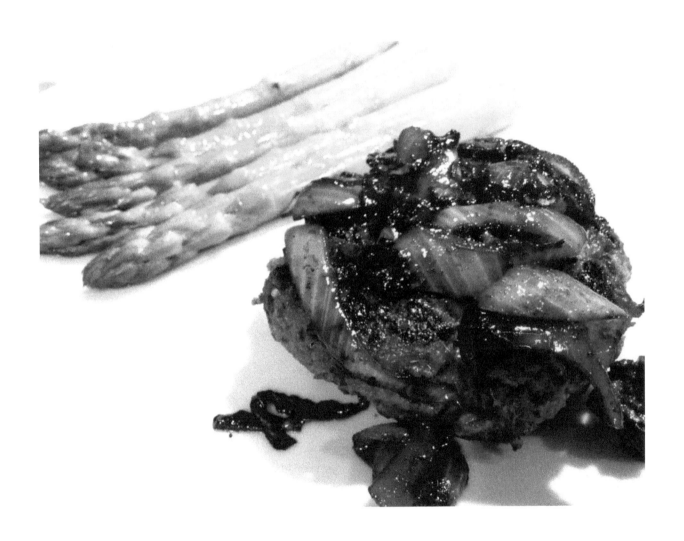

# Desserts

# PALEO CHOCOLATE PEPPERMINT CHIA SMOOTHIE

You can definitely enjoy the taste of chocolate through the peppermint chia smoothie.

MAKES 2 SERVING/ TOTAL TIME 10 MINUTE

## INGREDIENTS

2 Bananas (frozen)

2 tbsp Unsweetened cocoa powder

1 tbsp Chia seeds

1/2 tsp Peppermint extract

1 cup Almond milk

## METHOD

### STEP 1

Put all of the ingredients in a blender and blend until smooth and creamy. Serve immediately.

**NUTRITION VALUE**

498 Kcal, 20g fat,
3.9g fiber, 21.7g protein, 14.9g carbs.

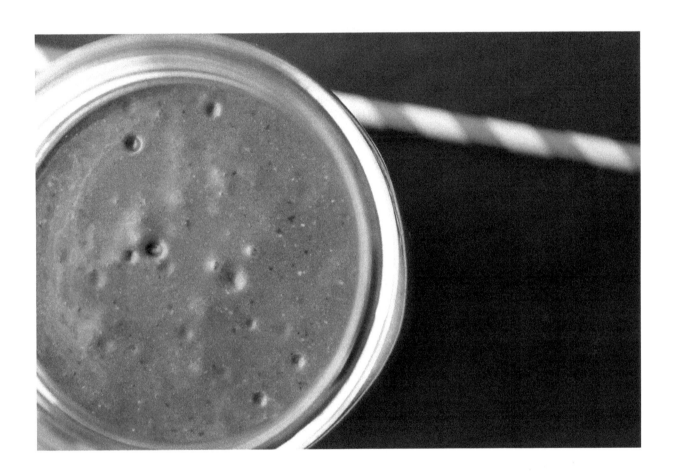

# BAKED APPLES

With only three ingredients you can create a comforting dessert that will help satisfy any sweet tooth—guilt-free

MAKES 2 SERVING/ TOTAL TIME 20 MINUTE

## INGREDIENTS

2 Apples (cored and quartered)

1 tbsp Ground cinnamon

1 tbsp Ghee

## METHOD

**STEP 1**

Preheat the oven to 350 degrees F.

Place the apples in an aluminum foil pouch. Sprinkle with cinnamon and add the ghee.

Close the pouch tightly.

**STEP 2**

Place in the oven and cook for 15 to 17 minutes, or until done.

Carefully open the pouch and serve.

| NUTRITION VALUE | 70 cal, 7g fat, 4g fiber, 11.3g protein, 7g carbs. |
|---|---|

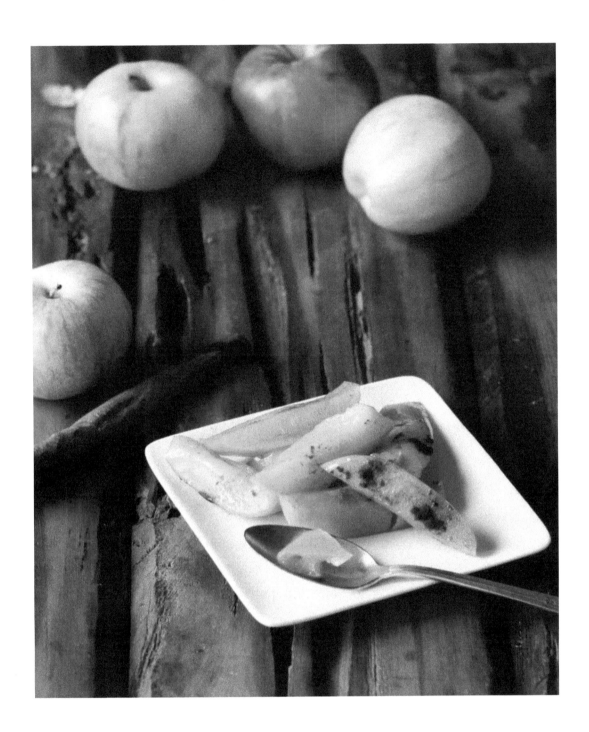

# COOKIE DOUGH TRUFFLES

The cookie dough is completely gluten-free and egg-free.

MAKES 1 SERVING/ TOTAL TIME 10 MINUTE

## INGREDIENTS

1 cup Almond flour

Pinch of sea salt

1 tbsp Coconut oil (melted)

1 tbsp Maple syrup

1 tsp Almond milk

1/2 tsp vanilla extract

2-3 tbsp Mini dark chocolate chips

## METHOD

**STEP 1**

Stir the almond flour and salt together in a medium bowl. Add the coconut oil, maple syrup, almond milk, and vanilla and stir well to combine.

Fold in the chocolate chips.

Using your hands, roll out the dough into a dozen small balls and set onto a plate.

**STEP 2**

Place in the refrigerator for 30 minutes.

Prepare a baking sheet with parchment paper.

Place the dark chocolate into a microwave-safe bowl and melt in the microwave.

Remove the cookie dough balls from the refrigerator.

Use a spoon to carefully dip each ball into the melted chocolate and then place onto the parchment paper.

Move the baking sheet into the freezer for 30 minutes to let the chocolate harden.

Store in the refrigerator.

**NUTRITION VALUE**

435 Cal, 20g fat, 7g saturated fat, 8g fiber, 21g protein, 14.9g carbs.

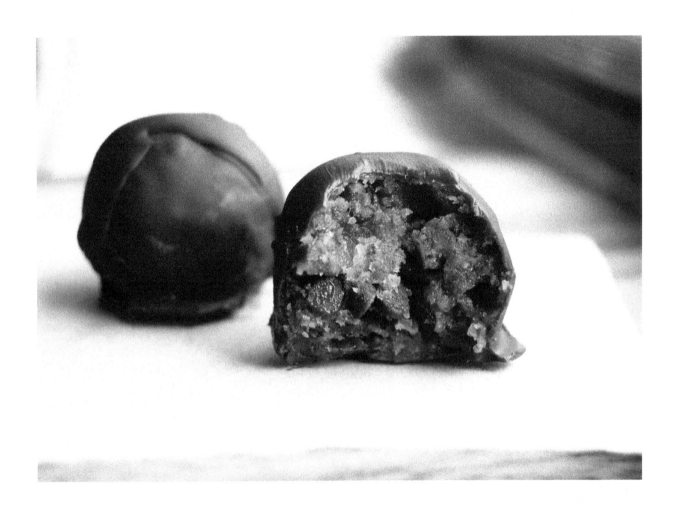

# MEXICAN CHOCOLATE MOUSSE

Silky and rich, this chocolate mousse takes only minutes to make and no cooking is required.

MAKES 4 SERVING/ TOTAL TIME 30 MINUTE

## INGREDIENTS

2 Ripe avocados

1 cup Coconut milk

1/2 cup Unsweetened cocoa powder

1/2 cup Honey

2 tsp Vanilla extract

2 tsp Cinnamon

1/2 tsp Ground ancho chile

## METHOD

**STEP 1**

Combine all of the ingredients together in a blender or food processor and process until smooth.

Adjust honey to taste.

Refrigerate for at least one hour before serving.

**NUTRITION VALUE**

275 Cal, 15g fat, 11g saturated fat, 11g fiber, 20g protein, 14g carbs.

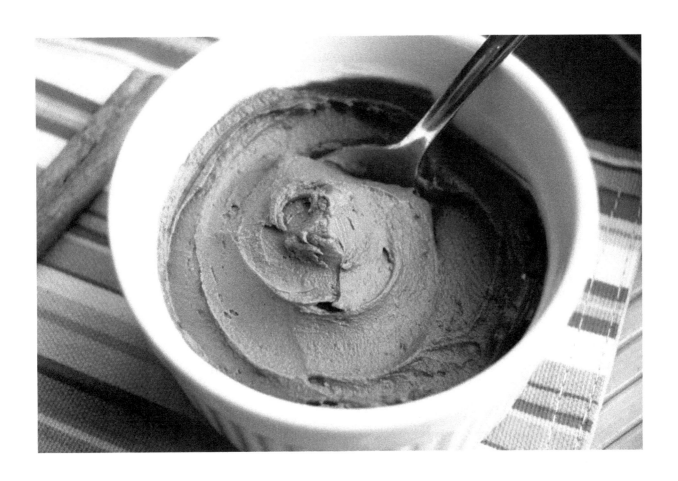

# DOUBLE CHOCOLATE BROWNIES

These fudgy brownies are decadent and delicious. They are very easy to make and don't require a ton of extra ingredients.

MAKES 9 SERVING/ TOTAL TIME 40 MINUTE

## INGREDIENTS

1/4 cup plus 3 tbsp Coconut flour

1/2 cup 100% Cocoa powder

1/2 cup plus 2 tbsp Ghee (substitute coconut oil, melted)

3 Eggs

3/4 cup Honey (agave)

2 tsp Vanilla extract

1/4 cup Paleo-friendly chocolate chips (chopped into chunks)

## METHOD

**STEP 1**

Preheat oven to 350 degrees F.

Grease an 8 x 8 baking sheet.

In a large, bowl whisk together the coconut flour and cocoa powder.

Add the melted ghee (or coconut oil), eggs, honey, and vanilla extract. Mix until well combined. Allow to sit for 5 minutes, the coconut flour will absorb the liquid and a batter will form.

**STEP 2**

Fold in the chocolate chips.

Spoon the batter into the greased baking sheet.

Bake for 30 to 40 minutes or until a toothpick comes out of the center clean.

Remove from the oven and allow to cool before serving.

**NUTRITION VALUE**

435 Cal, 20g fat, 7g saturated fat, 8g fiber, 21g protein, 14.9g carbs.

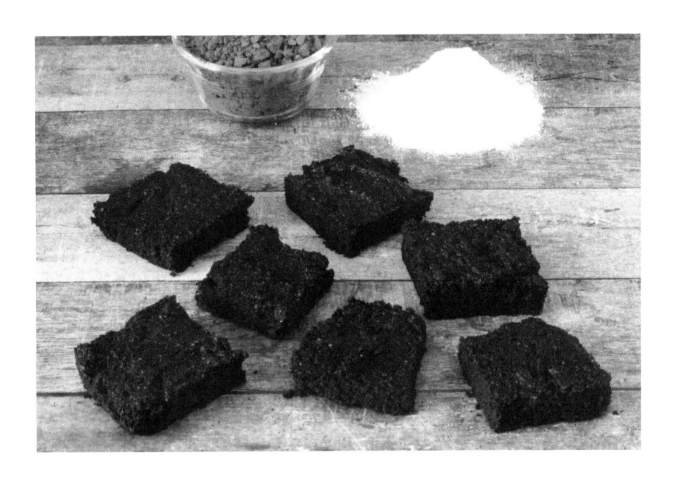

# PALEO MINT BROWNIES

Mint and chocolate are two ingredients that are often paired together and for good reason.

MAKES 2 SERVING/ TOTAL TIME30 MINUTE

## INGREDIENTS

1 cup Almond butter

1/3 cup Honey

1 Egg

2 tbsp Coconut oil (melted)

1 tsp Peppermint extract

1/4 cup Unsweetened cocoa powder

1/2 tsp Baking soda

Pinch of salt

Coconut oil spray

## METHOD

### STEP 1

Preheat the oven to 325 degrees F.

Place the almond butter, honey, egg, coconut oil, and peppermint extract into a large bowl.

Use a hand blender to combine until smooth.

### STEP 2

Mix in the cocoa powder, baking soda, and salt.

Prepare an 8x8-inch baking pan with coconut oil spray.

Spoon the batter into the pan and bake for 18-20 minutes, until a toothpick inserted into the center comes out clean.

**NUTRITION VALUE**

530 Cal, 20g fat, 11g saturated fat, 7g fiber, 21g protein, 14g carbs.

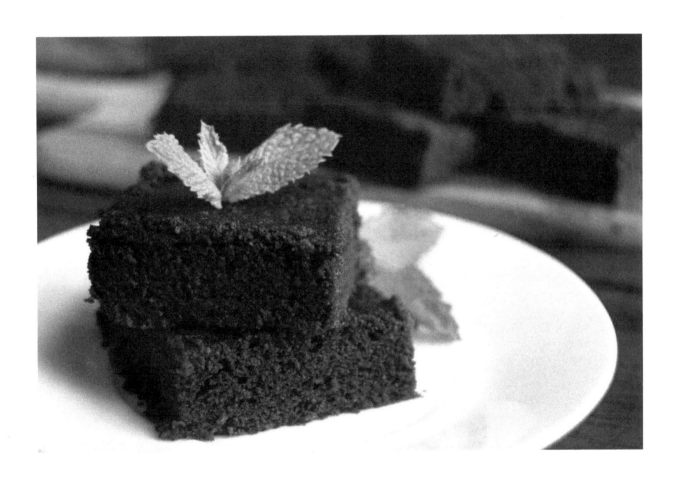

# Snacks

# MINT CHIP FREEZER BARS

This easy no-bake recipe is so pretty and delicious that it'll make it look like you spent hours slaving away in the kitchen!

MAKES 2 SERVING/ TOTAL TIME 20 MINUTE

## INGREDIENTS

Mint

1 Ripe avocado (large)

1/4 c Honey

6 tbsp Coconut oil (melted)

1.5 c Unsweetened coconut flakes (shredded)

1/2 tsp Mint extract

Pinch of sea salt

Chocolate

1/4 c Coconut oil (melted)

2 tbsp Honey

1/4 c Dark cocoa powder (unsweetened)

1/2 tsp Mint extract

Pinch of sea salt

## METHOD

In a powerful blender or food processor, mix together all ingredients for the mint layer until creamy.
Carefully pour the mixture into the 9x9 baking pan. Refrigerate for 15 minutes or until solid.
Meanwhile, melt the coconut oil for the chocolate topping in a small saucepan.
To avoid ending up with chunks, use a sifter to sift the cocoa powder into the coconut oil and honey mixture, stirring frequently.
Add mint extract and a pinch of sea salt and continue to stir well. The honey and the oil don't like to mix, so the constant stirring is necessary to keep them well combined and evenly distributed. Set aside the warm chocolate mixture and retrieve the 9x9 pan from the fridge.
Carefully pour the chocolate layer on top of the mint layer and turn the edges of the pan to evenly distribute the chocolate across the top. Refrigerate for another 20-30 minutes or until completely hardened before serving.
Gently flip it over and cut into bars. Store in the fridge or freezer and garnish with fresh mint leaves, if desired.

## NUTRITION VALUE

418 Cal, 8.7g fat, 1.9g saturated fat, 13.6g fiber, 20g protein, 14g carbs.

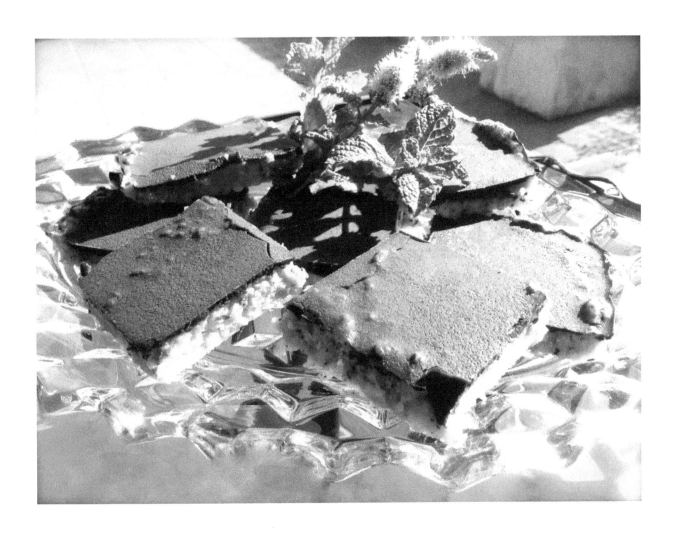

# CRUNCHY PLANTAIN CHIPS

These are so tasty you'll wish that you'd made a double batch! Enjoy with **Paleo Chocolate Chili**, Mango Pico de Gallo, **guacamole**, or plain for road trips!

MAKES 1 SERVING/ TOTAL TIME 10 MINUTE

## INGREDIENTS

2 Green plantains

Juice from 1 lime (about 1 tbsp)

1 tbsp Coconut oil

Sprinkle of garlic powder

Sea salt (to taste)

## METHOD

**STEP 1**

1Preheat oven to 400 degrees.

Peel and slice plantains as thinly as possible (be very careful) using a mandolin or a sharp knife. Slice them either lengthwise or round.

Add plantain slices to a parchment-covered baking sheet.

**STEP 2**

Drizzle with coconut oil and lime juice. Sprinkle with seasonings and salt to taste.

Bake for 20-25 minutes, flipping halfway through.

Eat immediately with Paleo Chocolate Chili or store in an airtight container to keep them crisp.

**NUTRITION VALUE**

331 Kcal, 20g fat, 5g fiber, 22g protein, 13g carbs.

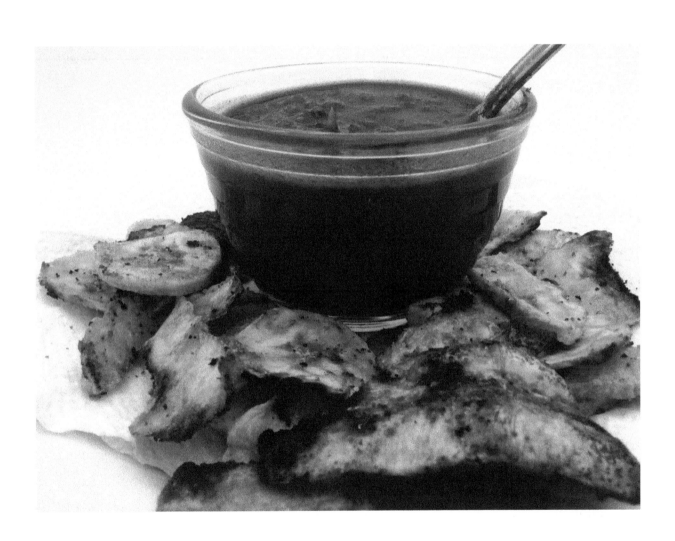

# BREADED CHICKEN STRIPS WITH DIJON HONEY MUSTARD DIPPING SAUCE

This recipe is for the new ultimate **fast-food** favorite for kids and adults alike!

MAKES 4 SERVING/ TOTAL TIME 25 MINUTE

## INGREDIENTS

4 Boneless (skinless chicken breasts)

2 Eggs (large)

1 1/2 c Almond flour

1/2 c Arrowroot powder

1/2 tsp plus 1/8 tsp. Sea salt

1/2 tsp Fresh ground black pepper

1/2 tsp Garlic powder (opt. seasoning)

1/2 tsp Onion powder (opt. seasoning)

1/2 tsp Paprika (opt. seasoning)

3-4 tbsp Ghee (or coconut oil)

3/4 c Paleo-friendly mayonnaise

1/4 c Dijon mustard

1 Garlic clove (minced)

3 tbsp Honey

## METHOD

Slice each chicken breast length-wise into 3-4 (1-inch) strips. In a shallow dish, whisk together the two eggs. Set aside. In a medium-sized mixing bowl combine the almond flour, arrowroot powder, ½ tsp. sea salt, ¼ tsp. black pepper, garlic powder, onion powder, and the paprika (opt.).

One by one, dip the chicken strips into the egg mixture, pausing above the mixture to let any excess egg drip off, and then dredging each strip through the almond flour mixture, making sure to coat all sides thoroughly. Place the strips onto a wire cooling rack while you finish coating the rest. Heat the ghee or coconut oil in a large skillet over medium-high heat. Place the strips in the pan and cook for about 4-5 minutes on each side prepare the Dijon Honey Mustard Dipping Sauce. To do so, in a medium-sized mixing bowl , combine the mayonnaise, Dijon mustard, minced garlic, honey, the remaining 1/8 tsp. sea salt, and the ¼ tsp. black pepper. Chill in the refrigerator until ready to serve.

| NUTRITION VALUE | 952 Cal, 20g fat, 13g saturated fat, 13.6g fiber, 20g protein, 14g carbs. |
|---|---|

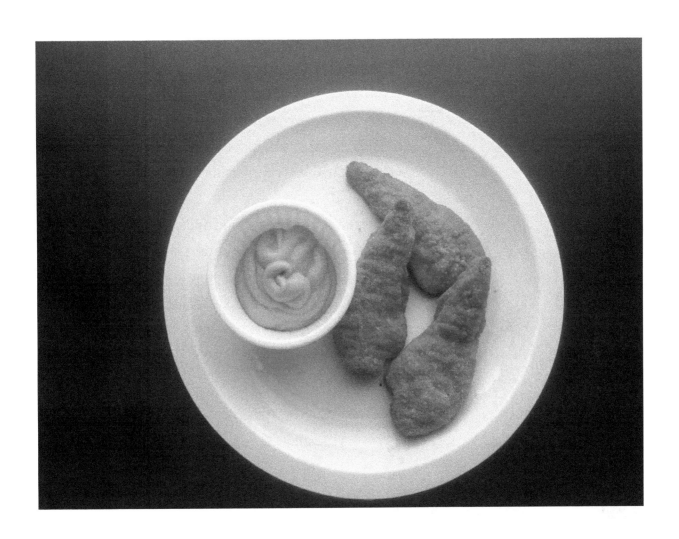

# SCRUMMY PRIMAL TORTILLAS

Tortillas in this cuisine is made up of finely grounded sweet potato.

## INGREDIENTS

2 Eggs

1 tbsp Grass fed butter (melted (primal))

1/2 c Sweet potato (mashed)

1 1/4 c Arrowroot powder

1/2 c Ground flax

1 c Water

1/2 tsp Sea salt

## METHOD

### STEP 1

Mix together melted butter, eggs, and sweet potato.
Note: I used a submersion blender to make it easier and to ensure a nice, smooth consistency.
Stir in arrowroot powder, the flax, and the sea salt.
Add in water and mix well. The mixture will have the consistency of runny pancake batter.

### STEP 2

Heat a skillet on medium and carefully pour 1/4 c of the batter into the middle of the skillet.
The tortillas are done on one side once they start to bubble in the middle like pancakes. Flip them over and cook the other side for about 30 seconds to 1 minute.
Set the cooked tortilla aside to cool and do it again!

## NUTRITION VALUE

382 Cal, 14g fat, 1.9g saturated fat, 8g fiber, 21g protein, 14g carbs.

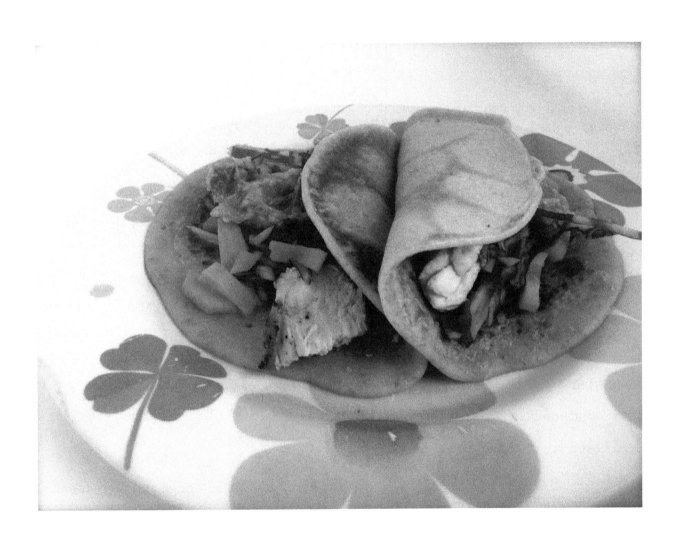

# GARLIC HERB BISCUITS

These tasty little primal nuggets are so delicious and comforting, you'll be in danger of overindulging! Serve them hot and fresh out of the oven as a snack or as a side for any special occasion meal.

MAKES 4 SERVING/ TOTAL TIME 30 MINUTE

## INGREDIENTS

1/2 c Water

1/2 c Grass fed butter (or coconut oil, primal not paleo)

1/2 tsp Sea salt

2 tbsp Apple cider vinegar

1/2 c Arrowroot powder

1 c Coconut flour

1/2 tsp Baking soda

1/2 tsp Baking powder

2 Eggs

For glazing

1 tsp Garlic powder

1 tsp Rosemary (dried)

2 tsp Grass fed butter (melted, or coconut oil -primal not paleo)

## METHOD

**STEP 1**

Preheat oven to 350.

In a medium saucepan, melt butter on low or add coconut oil. Then add water, salt, and vinegar. Turn up heat and bring to a boil. Remove pan from heat as soon as you see the mixture begin to boil.

Add the arrowroot powder and mix well. It will gel slightly. This is to be expected.

Add baking soda and powder and mix well. The reaction between the baking soda and vinegar will cause it to foam and rise slightly. This is normal.

Next, add in half of the coconut flour and mix it as well as you can. This is where the dough will start to get slightly dry. Don't panic. Wait to add the eggs in until the dough cools off a little,

**STEP 2**

Form 2-inch balls with the dough and place them on a parchment-lined baking sheet.

Brush balls with melted butter or coconut oil and top with garlic powder and rosemary.

Bake for 25 minutes or until slightly browned.

| NUTRITION VALUE | 262 Cal, 7g fat, 7g saturated fat, 28g fiber, 21g protein, 13g carbs. |
|---|---|

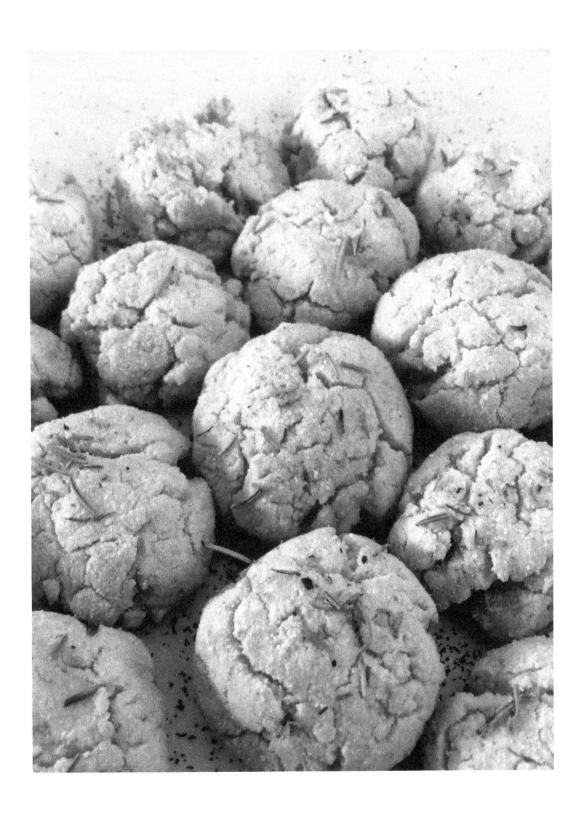

# CRUNCHY ALMOND BISCOTTI

Gluten-free biscotti are not difficult to make but they do take a bit of time to prepare.

MAKES 2 SERVING/ TOTAL TIME 1 HOUR

## INGREDIENTS

1 3/4 cups Almond flour

1/4 cup Coconut flour

1/2 tsp Baking soda

Pinch of salt

1/4 cup Honey

1 tsp Almond extract

1/4 cup Slivered almonds

## METHOD

**STEP 1**

Preheat the oven to 350 degrees F.

Stir together the almond flour, coconut flour, baking soda, and salt in a large bowl.

Add the honey and almond extract and stir to combine.

Fold in the slivered almonds.

Prepare a baking sheet with parchment paper.

Shape the dough into a log on the parchment paper.

Bake for 15 minutes or until lightly golden.

**STEP 2**

Let cool for one hour.

Reheat the oven to 250 degrees F.

Slice the biscotti into long thin pieces and bake for 15 minutes more.

Turn off the oven and crack open the door, letting the biscotti cool for one hour in the oven before serving.

## NUTRITION VALUE

796 Cal, 18.9g fat, 6g saturated fat, 21g fiber, 28g protein, 14g carbs.

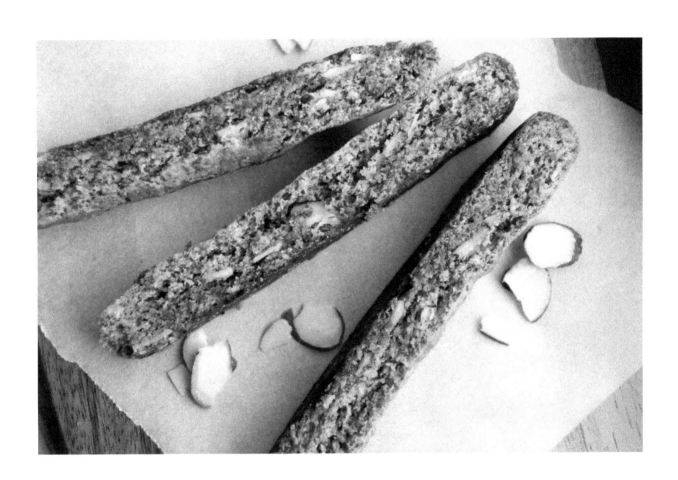

# GRAIN-FREE HONEY AND APRICOT PALEO GRANOLA

This recipe is for a Grain-Free Honey And Apricot Paleo Granola.

MAKES 4 SERVING/ TOTAL TIME 30 MINUTE

## INGREDIENTS

1 cup Almonds

1/2 cup Macadamia nuts

1/3 cup Unsweetened coconut flakes

1/4 cup Pumpkin seeds (shelled)

1/4 cup Coconut oil

3 tbsp Honey

1 tsp Vanilla extract

1/3 cup Apricots (dried, finely diced)

1/2 tsp Salt

## METHOD

### STEP 1

Preheat the oven to 300 degrees F.

Line a baking sheet with parchment paper.

Place the almonds, macadamia nuts, coconut flakes, and pumpkin seeds into a blender and pulse a few times to make smaller pieces.

Add the coconut oil, honey, and vanilla to a microwave-safe bowl.

### STEP 2

Heat in the microwave for 45 seconds.

Remove from the microwave and stir in the nut mixture, tossing well to thoroughly coat.

Stir in the apricots and salt.

Spread the granola onto the prepared baking sheet in an even layer and bake for 20 minutes or until lightly browned.

Allow to cool for 10 minutes before breaking into large pieces.

| NUTRITION VALUE | 822 Cal, 19g fat, 1.9g saturated fat, 10g fiber, 20g protein, 13g carbs. |
|---|---|

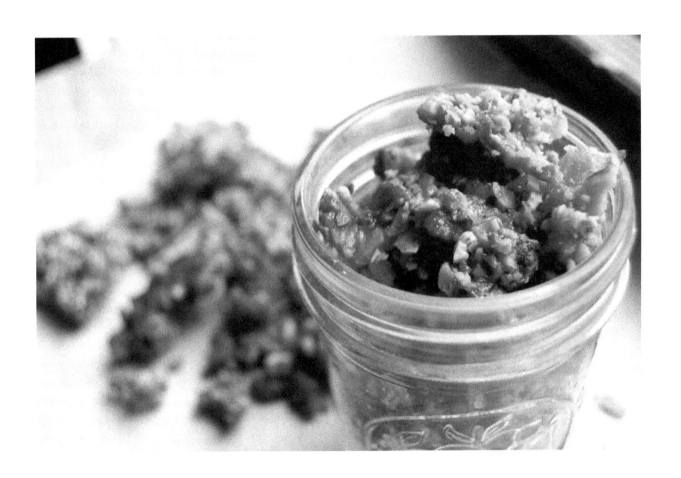

# MANGO GINGER SMOOTHIE

We recommend trying it mid-morning, to keep you awake while you work away.

MAKES 1 SERVING/ TOTAL TIME 10 MINUTE

## INGREDIENTS

1 cup Spinach

2 cups Water

1 Cucumber (peeled)

1 inch Ginger root

3 cups Mango (diced)

Juice from 1 lemon

## METHOD
### STEP 1
Combine all ingredients in a blender and pulse until smooth.

**NUTRITION VALUE**

129 Cal, 1g fat, 0.2g saturated fat, 5g fiber, 3g protein, 32g carbs.

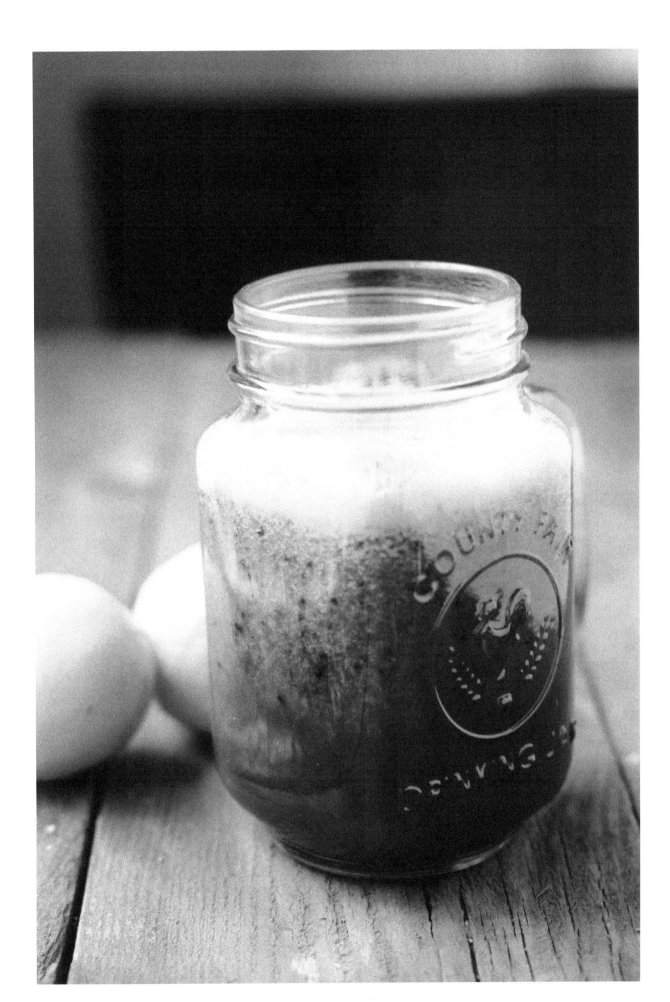

# ALMOND CANTALOUPE SMOOTHIE

Almond milk brings a creamy and nutty flavor to this smoothie.

MAKES 1 SERVING/ TOTAL TIME 10 MINUTE

## INGREDIENTS

2 cups Spinach

1 cup Almond milk (unsweetened)

1/2 Cantaloupe (ripe and rind removed)

1 cup Mixed berries

1/2 cup Water

1/2 Ice

## METHOD
### STEP 1
Combine all ingredients in a blender and pulse until smooth.

**NUTRITION VALUE**

69 Cal, 1g fat, 0.9g saturated fat, 4g fiber, 4g protein, 13g carbs.

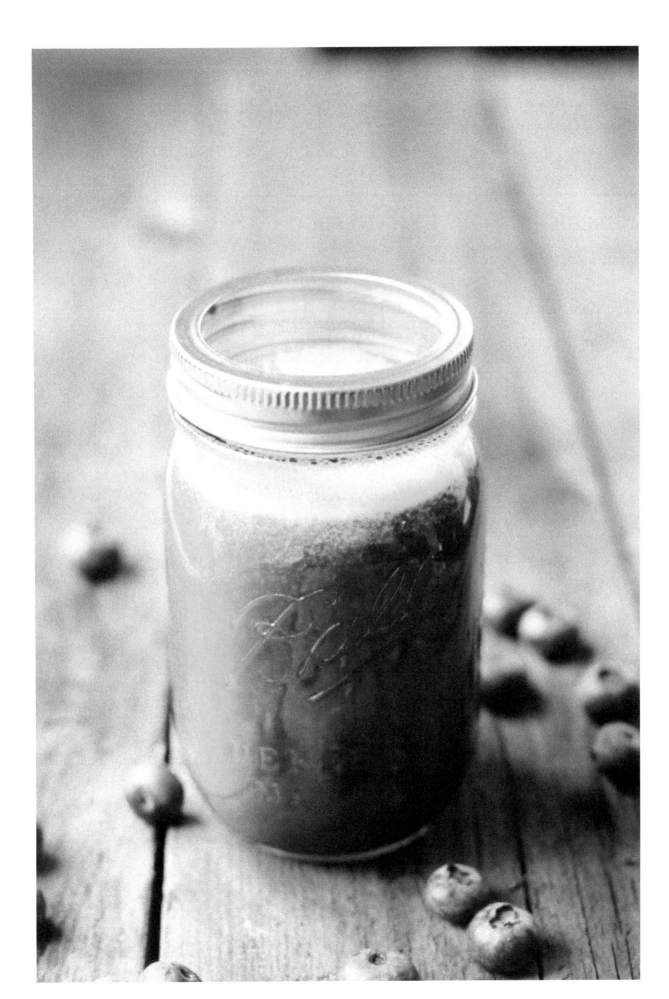

# FRESH MANGO SALSA

Dips and dressings are ideal for spicing up meat but the problem is that paleo dressings are hard to find.

## INGREDIENTS

1 Ripe mango, (large, cut into chunks (about 1 c))

1/2 c Tomatoes (diced)

1/2 c Onion (diced)

1/2 c Fresh cilantro (roughly chopped)

2 tbsp Juice from 2 limes

Sea salt and fresh ground pepper (to taste)

## METHOD

**STEP 1**

Mix diced mango, tomatoes, onion, and fresh cilantro together in a medium bowl.

Juice limes over diced salsa.

Add sea salt and pepper to taste.

Mix well, serve, and enjoy!

**NUTRITION VALUE**

27 Cal, 0.2g fat, 0.03g saturated fat, 2g fiber, 1g protein, 6g carbs.

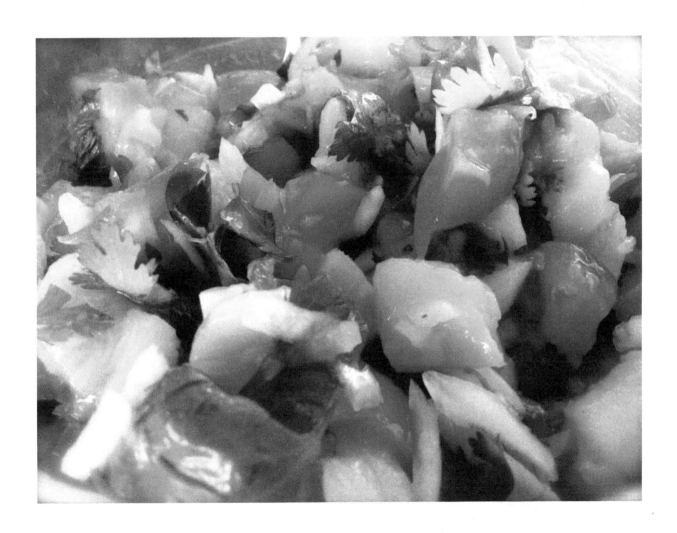

# VERY BERRY SMOOTHIE

Mix and match your favorites, blend them up, add some kiwi, and your taste buds won't know what's happened to them.

MAKES 1 SERVING/ TOTAL TIME 10 MINUTE

## INGREDIENTS

2 cups Spinach

2 cups Water

2 cup Mixed berries

1 Bananas (frozen)

1 Kiwi (peeled)

2 cups Water

## METHOD
### STEP 1

Combine all ingredients in a blender and pulse until smooth.

**NUTRITION VALUE**

82 Cal, 0.5g fat, 0.1g saturated fat, 5g fiber, 4g protein, 17g carbs.

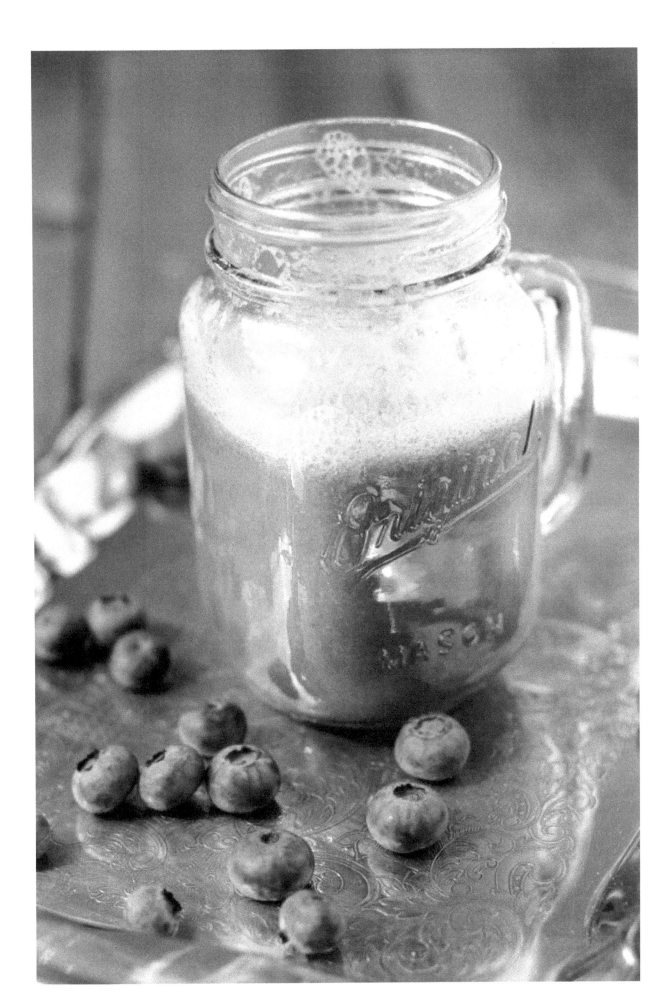

CPSIA information can be obtained
at www.ICGtesting.com
Printed in the USA
LVHW010814010621
689026LV00011B/1398